Self-Assessment Colour Review
Cattle and Sheep Medicine

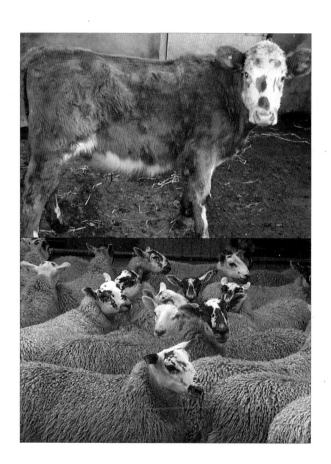

Self-Assessment Colour Review

Cattle and Sheep Medicine

Philip R Scott
BVM&S, MPhil, DVM&S, DSHP, FRCVS,
DiplECSRHM, DiplECBHM, FHEA
Royal (Dick) School of Veterinary Studies
Easter Bush Veterinary Centre
Easter Bush, Nr Roslin, Midlothian, UK

MANSON PUBLISHING/THE VETERINARY PRESS

Contents

Copyright © 2010 Manson Publishing Ltd
ISBN: 978-1-84076-126-9

A CIP catalogue record for this book is available from the British Library.

For full details of all Manson Publishing Ltd titles please write to:
Manson Publishing Ltd, 73 Corringham Road, London NW11 7DL, UK.
Tel: +44(0)20 8905 5150
Fax: +44(0)20 8201 9233
Website: www.mansonpublishing.com

Commissioning editor: Jill Northcott
Project manager: Paul Bennett
Copy editor: Joanna Brocklesby
Design and layout: Cathy Martin
Colour reproduction: Tenon & Polert Colour Scanning Ltd, Hong Kong
Printed by: New Era Printing Company Ltd, Hong Kong

Preface

This book aims to present the essential facts of the most common ruminant diseases and conditions in a problem-based format. Clinical cases are not ordered in organ system, thereby mimicking the random presentation of cases during a busy round of calls in practice. The diagnosis and treatment regimens described herein are those used by the author over the past 30 years in commercial large animal practice in the UK; they acknowledge the time and financial restrictions in many situations but require no specialized facilities nor equipment. The book is designed for veterinary undergraduates during their clinical rotations, and for the recent graduate who encounters the occasional farm animal problem in mixed practice. All suggestions for further cases, comments, and suggestions will be gratefully received and acknowledged by the author.

Philip R Scott

Abbreviations

AGID	agar gel immunodiffusion	L3	third stage larva
AP	alkaline phosphatase	LDA	left-displaced abomasum
AST	aspartate aminotransferase	MD	mucosal disease
BCS	body condition score	ME	metabolizable energy
BP	British Pharmacopoeia	MJ	megajoules
BRSV	bovine respiratory syncytial virus	MVV	maedi-visna virus
		NEFA	nonesterified fatty acid
BUN	blood urea nitrogen	NSAID	nonsteroidal anti-inflammatory drug
BVD	bovine virus diarrhoea		
CFT	complement fixation test	OPP	ovine progressive pneumonia
CLA	caseous lymphadenitis		
CNS	central nervous system	OPT	ovine pregnancy toxaemia
CPD	contagious pustular dermatitis	PCV	packed cell volume
		PEM	polioencephalomalacia
CSF	cerebrospinal fluid	PGE	parasitic gastroenteritis
DM	dry matter	RBC	red blood cell
EAE	enzootic abortion of ewes	SPA	sheep pulmonary adenomatosis
EDTA	ethylenediamine tetra-acetic acid		
		WBC	white blood cell
ELISA	enzyme-linked immunosorbent assay	ZN	Ziehl-Neelsen (stain)
epg	eggs per gram		
EU	European Union		
FAT	fluorescent antibody test		
GGT	gamma glutamyltransferase		
GLDH	glutamate dehydrogenase		
IBR	infectious bovine rhinotracheitis		
IKC	infectious keratoconjunctivitis		

Classification of Cases: Cattle

Cardiac disease 7, 73, 91, 109

Eye disorders 88

Foreign bodies 62, 71, 82, 112

Foot disease 4, 8, 13, 21, 29, 77, 89

Gastrointestinal system 10, 20, 30, 33, 38, 51, 62, 71, 85, 107

Genitourinary system 46, 51, 53, 63, 70, 79, 86, 106

Husbandry 42, 55, 72, 99, 101

Iatrogenic disease 96

Infectious disease 12, 19, 31, 34, 47, 48, 50, 72, 76, 78, 93, 94, 106, 110

Lameness 5, 8, 11, 13, 21, 27, 28, 29, 45, 61, 77, 89, 108

Metabolic and electrolyte disturbance 30, 40, 44, 68, 81, 83, 85, 92

Musculoskeletal system 4, 5, 13, 16, 27, 37, 45

Neurological disease 50, 52, 87, 93, 100, 108, 110

Newborn calf 16, 76, 77, 93, 97, 101

Nutrition and feeding 1, 23, 54, 68, 80, 81, 92

Parasitic disease 2, 14, 20, 72

Parturition and pregnancy 25, 39, 41, 51, 52, 63, 86, 90, 98, 100, 102, 103, 104

Prevention of disease/injury 34, 95, 99, 101, 111

Respiratory disease 4, 36, 43, 47, 65

Skin disease 14, 22, 66, 74, 84

Surgical procedures 13, 32, 53, 55, 64, 69, 71

Toxins 1, 49

Trauma and fractures 11, 28, 46, 52, 58, 60, 75

Tumours 59, 88

Classification of Cases: Sheep

1 You are presented with two 15-month-old dairy heifers which have been housed for 2 weeks and fed the remains of last year's silage clamp before the new clamp is opened. The heifers are very weak and unable to rise (1a). The farmer had noted that one heifer in the group of 84 was unsteady on its hindlegs the previous evening. None of the other heifers show

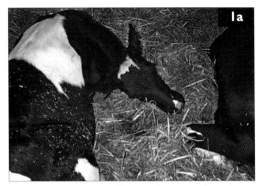

any abnormal clinical signs. Both heifers appear dull and depressed and are unable to rise. There is profound weakness of the limb muscles. The rectal temperature is normal for each heifer. The heifers do not eat but can swallow. There are ruminal movements but only scant mucus-coated faeces are passed.
i. What conditions would you suspect? (Most likely first.)
ii. What treatments would you administer?
iii. What control measures could be adopted?

2 A 3-year-old dairy heifer presents with 2 months' history of weight loss and diarrhoea despite anthelmintic treatment by the farmer. The heifer was purchased soon after calving 3 months ago and is yielding only 18 L/day. The rectal temperature is normal. No significant clinical signs are found except for profuse diarrhoea without blood or mucosal casts and poor body condition (2).

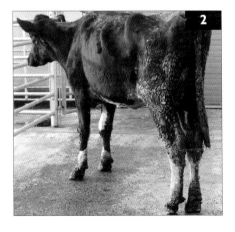

i. What conditions would you consider? (Most likely first.)
ii. Which further tests could be undertaken?
iii. What treatments would you recommend?
iv. What control measures must be adopted for introduced cattle?

1 i. The most likely conditions to consider include: botulism; lead poisoning; listeriosis; blackleg; recumbency and endotoxaemia associated with septicaemia.

There is no readily available diagnostic test for botulinum toxin. There was no access to poultry waste/carcasses, the most common source of botulinum toxin, but the farmer often shot a large number of feral pigeons in the shed that may

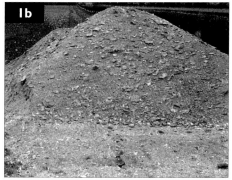

have resulted in carcass contamination of the clamp silage which was not sheeted.

ii. There is no specific treatment although cattle displaying only pelvic limb weakness may recover over 7–14 days. In this problem, one heifer deteriorated rapidly overnight (paralysis of tongue and masticatory muscles, head averted against chest) and was euthanased for welfare reasons. The other recumbent heifer was destroyed for welfare reasons 2 days later.

iii. To control this problem the old silage was discarded and the new silage pit opened. No further cases of botulism were reported in this group. Other control measures include preventing access to potentially contaminated feedstuffs especially poultry waste. Poultry manure is often used as a fertilizer applied directly to pasture (**1b**). Several recent outbreaks of botulism have been tentatively linked to feeding bakery waste to cattle.

2 i. The most likely conditions to consider include: Johne's disease (*Mycobacterium paratuberculosis*); chronic fasciolosis; persistent infection with BVD/MD virus; chronic salmonellosis; chronic bacterial infection leading to debility.

ii. Further tests include the ELISA test and faecal smear for Johne's disease, which were negative in this case. A faecal sample should be examined for parasite eggs, and an ELISA test can be carried out for liver fluke. In this case, a single fluke egg is seen on sedimentation; no strongyle eggs are detected by the modified McMaster method. The ELISA test for liver fluke is positive.

iii. Treatment could include triclabendazole or nitroxynil.

iv. All introduced cattle should be treated for intestinal parasites and fluke on arrival on the farm where appropriate. All cattle must be screened for BVD/MD virus status with seronegative animals checked for antigen. Vaccination against leptospirosis and IBR will depend upon the herd history but should be carefully considered. Single screening for chronic carrier status with *Salmonella dublin* is unreliable.

3 A 4-month-old Holstein bull calf presents with chronic severe bloat. The bull belongs to a group of 20 fattening cattle fed a high-production ration comprising *ad libitum* barley and protein balancer. The farmer has relieved the bloat five times over the previous week with an orogastric tube.

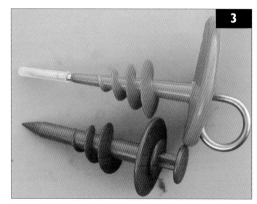

i. What are the options other than trocharization of the rumen (3)? List the advantages and disadvantages of the various methods.
ii. How would you insert the trochar?
iii. What is the prognosis?

4 Over a 4-week period, four of 12 dairy calves purchased directly from a single source at 2 weeks old have presented with septic pedal arthritis 4–6 weeks later, necessitating digit amputation (4). Other calves in the group have been treated several times for respiratory disease and are not growing well. The calves are housed in a large, well bedded straw pen and fed reconstituted milk substitute in a feed trough and *ad libitum* calf rearing pencils.

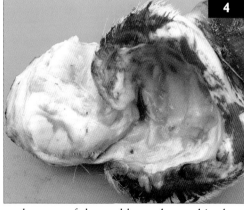

i. How would you investigate the causal agents of the problems observed in these calves?
ii. What are the possible causes?
iii. What treatments would you administer?
iv. What disease problem might be expected in the herd of origin?
v. What control measures would you recommend?

3 i. Trocharization: *Advantages* – quick therefore cheap. Granulation tissue seals the fistula within days of trochar removal. *Disadvantages* – the trochar may become dislodged and it then proves difficult to insert another. Spiral trochars are much more effective than straight trochars.

Make a semi-permanent rumen fistula: *Advantages* – granulation tissue seals the fistula only after several months. *Disadvantages* – requires abdominal surgery taking approximately 20 minutes including preparation time, therefore it is the most costly option. Rumen liquor escapes on to the flank, which is irritant and unsightly.

ii. The trochar is more easily inserted in the bloated animal. The site chosen is the highest point midway between the last rib and wing of the ilium. The site is infiltrated with lidocaine, and a 4 cm skin incision is made. The trochar point is pushed through the muscle layers and rumen wall, then the trochar is screwed into the rumen wall. The gas is released slowly over 2–3 minutes. The trochar is fixed to the skin with nonabsorbable sutures.

iii. Antibiotic therapy is often administered following surgery to treat possible infections affecting the forestomachs. Where available, transfaunation from a healthy animal is helpful. The protein content of the ration should be checked, ensuring a minimum of 16% crude protein and adequate long fibre. The prognosis is generally poor because chronic recurrent bloat is commonly caused by vagal indigestion.

4 i. Investigations could include arthrocentesis before antibiotic therapy and culture of synovial membrane collected after digit amputation. Bronchoalveolar lavage for BRSV is too late in the disease course. Bacteriological culture of bronchoalveolar lavage fluid could be undertaken but this is of doubtful benefit. Paired serology to determine respiratory virus involvement and BVD/MD status would be influenced by maternally derived antibody.

ii. The most likely conditions to consider include: septic joint – *Salmonella* spp. particularly *S. dublin* and *S. typhimurium* in this age range; respiratory disease – bacterial pneumonia following respiratory viral infection; persistently infected BVD/MD calf in the group causing transient infection in the other calves.

Culture of synovial membrane after digit amputation yields *S. dublin*.

iii. The response to parenteral antibiotic therapy for joint infections (usually florfenicol), and respiratory disease caused by *S. dublin*, is poor. Joint lavage necessitates general anaesthesia and often a second flush 3–5 days later. Digit amputation in the present situation gives good results and is the most economic option.

iv. Abortion at 5–7 months is a feature of herds with endemic *S. dublin* infection.

v. Control measures include stopping purchase of calves from this source. If the farmer is contracted to do so, the calves should be vaccinated at the source farm.

5 A 6-year-old Limousin bull presented with sudden onset lameness 12 months previously. A traumatic aetiology was suspected and the bull rested but he remains stiff on the right hindleg with an obvious bony swelling now apparent on the medial aspect of the right hock (5). The bull is 3/10 lame at the walk. The right hock joint capsule is not thickened nor is there any joint effusion. The bony swelling is smooth and not painful. There are no other swollen joints.

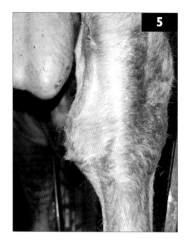

i. What conditions would you consider? (Most likely first.)
ii. What further examinations would you recommend?
iii. What advice would you offer?

6 You are presented with a 2-year-old Charolais bull which has had difficulty grazing for the past 4 days, caused by the inability to close his mouth fully. The bull appears dull and depressed but is aware of your presence and the confines of his new surroundings following housing. The bull appears slightly ataxic when walking to the cattle stocks.

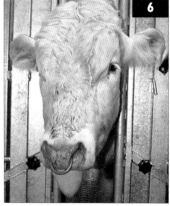

The bull's rectal temperature is 40.5°C (104.9°F). There is a normal menace response in both eyes but the pupillary light reflexes are absent. There is also bilateral dorsal strabismus but no nystagmus. There is exophthalmos of the right eye. There is bilateral paralysis of the masticatory muscles with impaction of roughage in the cheeks. There is passive protusion of the tongue which can be withdrawn upon stimulation (6). The bull experiences difficulty swallowing but is able to eat concentrates when the feed container is raised to shoulder height. There is no obvious head tilt. Auscultation of the chest fails to reveal any abnormal lung sounds. There is a marked bradycardia (42 beats per minute). There are normal ruminal contractions.

i. What conditions would you consider? (Most likely first.)
ii. What's your provisional diagnosis? (Give a neurological justification.)
iii. What treatment(s) would you administer?
iv. What control measures would you recommend?

5, 6: Answers

5 i. The most likely conditions to consider include: osteophyte deposition involving the tarsometatarsal joint (bone spavin); osteochondritis dissecans; trauma to the hock joint/ligamentous damage causing osteoarthritis.

ii. Radiography of right hock (left hock radiographs taken for comparison) reveals extensive new bone deposition involving the tarsometatarsal joint. Ultra-sonographic examination of the right hock joint reveals no thickening of the joint capsule or joint effusion.

iii. The tarsometatarsal joint is a low motion joint and therefore ankylosis should not limit locomotion except that great strain will be placed on this joint during mounting at service. There are a number of options; leave for another 6 months and radiograph again, turn the bull out with half the usual number of cows (20) with the risk of possible fracture through the bridging callus, or cull the bull. The third option was chosen (value of bull as cull animal representing almost 50% of the purchase price of a replacement); however, this may not be the correct option as there are no published studies on this type of injury. The second option could work but is it worth the risk on animal welfare grounds?

6 i. The most likely conditions to consider include: basilar empyema (pituitary abscess); listeriosis; peripheral vestibular lesion; brain abscess; bovine spongiform encephalopathy; botulism; rabies.

ii. A diagnosis of basilar empyema is based on the clinical findings of multiple cranial nerve deficits, particularly bilateral cranial nerve deficits involving III and V, ataxia, and bradycardia.

Ataxia results from interruption of extrapyramidal motor nuclei in the brain stem by the expanding abscess. Extension into the retro-orbital rete would explain the exophthalmos of the right eye.

iii. Recovery of cattle from basilar empyema depends on early detection of illness by the farmer and aggressive antibiotic treatment. *Arcanobacterium pyogenes* is most commonly isolated from such cases and is susceptible to various antibiotics including penicillin, ceftiofur, erythromycin, and trimethoprim/sulphonamide.

Treatment involves 44,000 IU/kg procaine penicillin injected intramuscularly twice daily for 3 weeks. The clinical signs remained unchanged for 5 days, then the bull's appetite improved and he was able to eat silage without food material becoming impacted. The bull's demeanour also improved. This response should be judged against deterioration in clinical signs and death in untreated cases 7–10 days after clinical signs first appear. The bull made a full recovery.

iv. The insertion of bull rings is considered a major risk factor with resultant localized infection spreading haematogenously to the rete mirabile, the complex of blood capillaries surrounding the pituitary gland, giving rise to basilar empyema.

7 A 6-year-old Holstein cow presents with 3 weeks' history of poor
appetite, weight loss, and reduced
milk yield (7a). Treatment with
intramuscular injection of oxytetracycline for 4 consecutive days by the
farmer has effected no improvement.
The rectal temperature is marginally
elevated (39.2°C (102.6°F)). The
cow is dull and depressed, and walks
slowly. There is distension of the
jugular veins and accumulation of
oedema under the brisket and

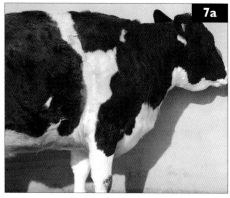

mandible which pits under digital pressure. The ocular and oral mucous
membranes are congested. The heart rate is 80 beats per minute but the heart
sounds are muffled on both sides of the chest. The respiratory rate is elevated to
40 breaths per minute with a slight abdominal component.
i. What conditions would you consider?
ii. Why is there oedema present?
iii. How could you confirm your provisional diagnosis?
iv. What treatment would you recommend?
v. What is the prognosis?

8 You are presented with a lame dairy cow
which has been 9/10 lame on the left foreleg
for the past 4 days. The cow is due to calve in
approximately 1 month and is at pasture with
a group of 12 other dry cows. Examination of
the leg fails to reveal any swelling, heat or pain.
The prescapular lymph node is of normal size.
The interdigital skin appears normal and
careful foot paring fails to reveal any abnormality. Examination of the dorsal hoof wall
reveals a small sandcrack (8). Application of
pressure over the sandcrack using hoof testers
elicits a painful reaction. Careful foot paring
releases an abscess.
i. What further treatments are indicated?
ii. What is the cause of such lesions?

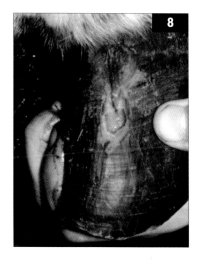

7 i. The most likely conditions to consider include: pericarditis; endocarditis; myocarditis/dilated cardiomyopathy; chronic suppurative respiratory disease; liver abscessation; pyelonephritis; lymphosarcoma involving the mediastinum and pericardium (enzootic bovine leucosis positive cows).

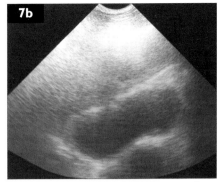

ii. In pericardial disease both cardiac filling and the ability of the ventricles and atria to clear the cardiac blood can be impaired. A gradual increase in pericardial pathology leads to a progression of this restrictive physiology and an impairment of normal diastolic filling of the heart. The resulting increases in intracardiac pressures can lead to right atrioventricular insufficiency and then to backward right-sided cardiac failure and increased venous pressure in the systemic circulation. Venous congestion results in vascular leakage causing oedema.

iii. Pericardial effusion can be readily demonstrated using a 5 MHz sector scanner and differentiated on appearance (effusion versus pus) (7b). Clinical pathology findings of leucocytosis (with left shift), increased fibrinogen, and increased serum globulin are nonspecific and could be present in many types of chronic bacterial infection.

iv. The bacterial flora present in bovine pericarditis is variable and may include single or mixed infections of staphylococci, streptococci, *Arcanobacterium*, *Escherichia coli*, and anaerobes. However, antibiotic therapy will not resolve this infection.

v. The prognosis is hopeless in cases of suppurative pericarditis and this cow should be destroyed for welfare reasons.

8 i. No bandage is necessary because the laminae are not exposed and there is no risk of exuberant granulation tissue formation. Antibiotic therapy is not indicated.

ii. Sandcracks result from a loss of continuity of horn fibres of the plantar hoof wall extending for a variable distance in the area between the coronet and the bottom of the wall. The aetiology is unknown but excessive drying out of the hoof horn during dry summer months or sudden excessive pressure from jumping and galloping has been suggested. This condition is more commonly seen in the Galloway breed and their crosses, suggesting a hereditary component.

9 You are presented with a collapsed 2-month-old beef calf (9). The rectal temperature is subnormal (38.1°C (100.6°F)). The eyes are markedly sunken and the skin tent is extended beyond 5 s, consistent with 7–10% dehydration. The ocular and oral mucous membranes are markedly congested. The heart rate is 120 beats per minute. The respiratory rate is elevated to 28 breaths per minute with a slight expiratory grunt. The abdomen is distended and palpation elicits a painful grunt.

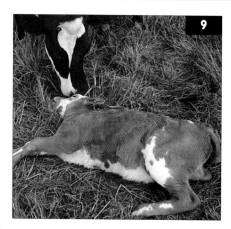

i. What conditions would you consider?
ii. How could you confirm your provisional diagnosis?
iii. What is the prognosis?
iv. What treatment would you recommend?
v. What control measures would you recommend?

10 A 5-year-old dairy cow presents with 6 weeks' history of increasing abdominal distension and loss of condition (10). The cow's appetite is poor and there are only scant hard faecal balls coated in mucus in the rectum. The cow has a roached-back appearance and an anxious expression. The abdomen is markedly distended and 'papple-shaped' (10 to 4 distension). The rectal temperature is normal. The pulse rate is 38 beats per minute. The force and rate of rumen contractions is increased to approximately three to four cycles per minute (normal rate is one cycle every 40 s or so). The withers pinch test (Williams' test) is negative.

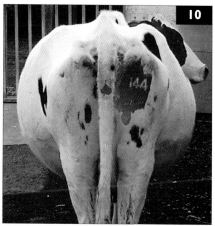

Passage of a stomach tube releases only a small amount of gas.
i. What conditions would you consider? (Most likely first.)
ii. How would you confirm your diagnosis?
iii. What actions/treatments would you recommend?

9, 10: Answers

9 i. The most likely conditions to consider include: abomasal perforation; clostridial enteritis; intestinal torsion; acute peritonitis; hairball causing obstruction to abomasal outflow; intussusception; necrotic enteritis; septicaemia; ruptured bladder/uroperitoneum.

ii. The clinical diagnosis could be supported by abdominocentesis, which would yield blood-tinged fluid. Ultrasonography may reveal several litres of fluid in the peritoneal cavity. Explorative laparotomy may be undertaken.

iii. The prognosis for abomasal perforation/acute septic peritonitis is hopeless despite early veterinary attention. Profound weakness, dehydration, injected mucous membranes, rapid pulse >100 beats per minute, and expiratory grunt are poor prognostic indicators.

iv. Symptomatic treatment comprises 2.2 mg/kg of flunixin meglumine injected intravenously. Five litres of isotonic saline are given intravenously over 1 hr (50 mL/kg). A further 5 L of isolec are infused over the next 3 hr. In this case a midline explorative laporotomy under xylazine (0.1 mg/kg intramuscularly) and ketamine (2–3 mg/kg intravenously) general anaesthesia revealed an abomasal perforation with contamination of the abdominal cavity. The calf was euthanased for welfare reasons.

v. Abomasal perforation through a single focal 1–2 cm diameter punctate ulcer occurs sporadically in 2–3-month-old beef calves. The cause of this sporadic condition has not been determined.

10 i. The most likely conditions to consider include: vagus indigestion; chronic bloat resulting from mediastinal mass, e.g. thymic lymphosarcoma or abscess; twin pregnancy/hydrops allantois; localized peritonitis; left-displaced abomasum; traumatic reticulitis.

ii. A diagnosis of vagus indigestion is based upon the clinical findings (rumen hypermotility, bradycardia, abdominal shape) and exclusion of other conditions. Localized peritonitis, often arising from traumatic reticulitis, is considered to be the most common cause of vagus indigestion. Ultrasonographic examination of the anterior abdomen using a 5 MHz sector scanner failed to detect any abdominal abscess. Abdominocentesis yielded a small quantity of straw-coloured peritoneal fluid with a low protein concentration and low cell count comprised mainly of lymphocytes (normal values).

iii. The prognosis in this cow was considered to be very poor due to the chronicity and severity of the abdominal distension and the cow was euthanased for welfare reasons. While the lack of specific diagnosis is very frustrating there is nothing more that can be done and the animal's welfare is the most important factor.

11 A yearling pedigree Charolais heifer presents with 8/10 lameness affecting the left hindleg having gone suddenly lame 3 months previously. Initially the heifer had great difficulty rising but the severity of the lameness has reduced slightly although the animal spends much more time than normal lying down. There is extensive muscle atrophy of the left gluteal muscle mass (11a). There is normal anal tone and no

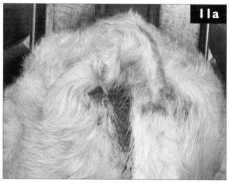

bladder atony/distension. The tail is pulled toward the unaffected side caused by atrophy of muscles of the affected side. There is increased extension of the right hind fetlock joint with outward rotation of the distal limb caused by disproportionate weightbearing. Palpation of the left limb fails to reveal any abnormality involving, or distal to, the left stifle joint. Lateral movement of the hindquarters produces a slight clunking sensation in the left hip region.
i. What conditions would you consider?
ii. How could you confirm your diagnosis?
iii. What action would you take?

12 A 6-year-old Holstein cow, which calved 36 hr earlier, is presented in sternal recumbency (12), profoundly depressed, dehydrated, afebrile (38.5°C (101.3°F)), with toxic mucous membranes, an elevated heart rate of 96 beats per minute, and an increased respiratory rate (34 breaths per minute). The udder is soft but a pale, serum-like, secretion can be drawn from one quarter.
i. Which diseases would you consider? (Most likely first.)
ii. What treatments would you administer?
iii. What control measures could be adopted?

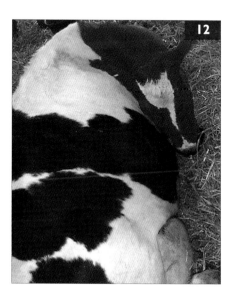

11 i. The most likely conditions to consider include: femoral fracture through the proximal growth plate; pelvic fracture involving the acetabulum; septic physitis leading to fracture through the proximal femoral growth plate; septic hip joint; dislocated hip; fracture of the femoral shaft. There is no evidence of hip dislocation. The pelvis appears symmetrical.

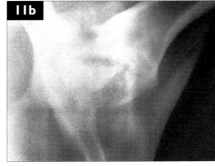

ii. The close proximity of the proximal growth plate to the hip joint and overlying muscle masses present problems with interpretation of ultrasound images. Radiography necessitates dorsal recumbency and either deep sedation or general anaesthesia and a powerful machine for cattle >200 kg.

iii. The heifer must be euthanased immediately even without radiographic confirmation of the fracture through the proximal femoral growth plate (this case). There is no condition listed above (i) that could reasonably be expected to resolve when the heifer is still severely lame 3 months after the event. This type of fracture is all too obvious following radiography (**11b**).

12 i. The most likely conditions to consider include: environmental (coliform) mastitis; hypocalcaemia; acute septic metritis; other infectious conditions causing toxaemia/endotoxaemia; trauma at parturition with either ruptured uterus/peritonitis or severe haemorrhage; botulism.

It may prove difficult to rule out the possible contribution of hypocalcaemia and many clinicians would elect to administer 400 mL of 40% calcium borogluconate slowly by the intravenous route while monitoring the heart rate.

ii. Treatment of endotoxic shock (coliform mastitis) includes intravenous injection of a NSAID, repeated 12 hr later. Hypertonic saline (7.2%) infusion at a dose rate of 5 mL/kg (3 L for 600 kg cow) over 5–7 minutes is achieved through a 13-gauge 10 cm jugular catheter. Access to 30–60 L of warm water, which may contain electrolytes, must be provided although not all cows drink; some clinicians recommend stomach tubing volumes up to 30–40 L. This cow made a full recovery.

Mastitis caused by *Streptococcus uberis* can present with many of the clinical features of coliform mastitis and it may prove prudent to administer a broad-spectrum antibiotic both parenterally and by intramammary infusion.

iii. Control measures include proper hygiene in the calving accommodation. Premilking teat dipping should be included in the parlour routine. Cows should be kept standing for 30 minutes after milking to enable complete teat sphincter contraction. Teat sealants should be used at drying-off. Use of J5 *Escherichia coli* core antigen vaccine could be considered.

13 A Limousin bull presents with severe (10/10) lameness of the left pelvic limb with marked muscle atrophy over the left hip. The left hindfoot is swollen with marked widening of the interdigital space. There is loss of hair and thinning of the skin extending all around the coronary band of the lateral claw extending proximally for 3 cm with a discharging sinus consistent with septic pedal arthritis.

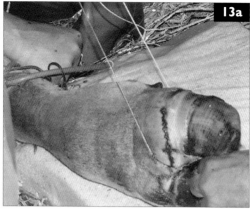

i. Describe the method of analgesia you would employ for the procedure illustrated here (13a)?
ii. How would you complete the procedure shown?

14 A group of beef cattle presents with 4 weeks' history of pruritus and extensive hair loss especially over the shoulder, neck, and ears (14). The cattle are frequently observed rubbing against walls and fence posts.

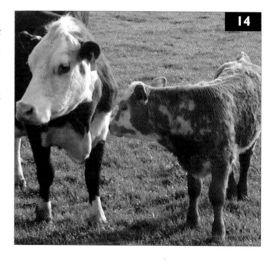

i. What conditions would you consider?
ii. Which further tests could be undertaken?
iii. What actions/treatments would you recommend?
iv. Are there any consequences of this problem?

13, 14: Answers

13 i. The procedure shown is digit amputation under intravenous regional anaesthesia. Flunixin meglumine (or other NSAID) is injected intravenously before surgery. A robust tourniquet is placed below the hock and 30–40 mL of 2% lidocaine solution is injected into the superficial vein running on the cranio-lateral aspect of the third metatarsal bone (butterfly catheter shown *in situ*). Analgesia is effective within 2 minutes.

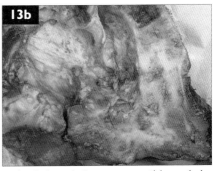

ii. The interdigital skin is incised as close to the infected tissue as possible and the incision extended for the full length of the interdigital space to a depth of 2 cm cranially increasing to 4 cm caudally. A length of embryotomy wire is introduced into the incision and the lateral digit removed at the level of mid P2 (wire at 15° to horizontal). A melolin dressing (or similar) is applied to the wound then cotton wool and a pressure bandage applied using Elastoplast (or similar). The dressing is changed after 4 days. The bull made a full recovery and is still in the herd 18 months later. A sagittal section through the amputated digit with P2 removed clearly shows the extent of infection and pathology within the distal interphalangeal joint (**13b**).

If infection in the deep flexor tendon sheath has extended above the amputation site, 10–15 cm of flexor tendon can be removed to effect drainage.

14 i. The most likely conditions to consider include: lice (pediculosis); forage mites; sarcoptic mange; chorioptic mange; ringworm (*Trichophyton* spp. infection).
ii. Inspection of the skin reveals extensive louse infestation. Microscopic examination of skin scraping reveals numerous chewing (round mouthparts; *Damalinia bovis*) and sucking lice (narrow and more pointed mouthparts; *Linognathus vituli*).
iii. Treatment options include pour-on organophosphorous or pyrethroid (e.g. cypermethrin) compounds that effect rapid improvement but may require re-treatment in 2–4 weeks. All in-contact cattle must be treated. Injectable avermectin products are not always wholly effective against chewing lice.

Pediculosis is widespread in all beef herds and routine treatment is recommended at housing. Interestingly, bulls are invariably more severely affected than cows.
iv. Disruption to grazing/feeding may cause reduced liveweight gain/loss of body condition in severe infestations, although very heavy burdens are more often a consequence rather than the cause of debility. Anaemia, as a consequence of severe infestations, is rare.

15 A 30-month-old Holstein heifer presents with 10 days' history of poor appetite and weight loss (15a). The heifer produced a live calf unaided 3 weeks previously and is yielding 16 L of milk per day. The heifer is dull and depressed. The rectal temperature is 39.2°C (102.6°F). The ocular and oral mucous membranes appear slightly congested. The heart rate is 86 beats per minute. The respiratory rate is 38

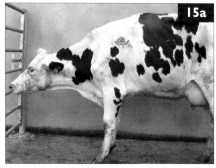

breaths per minute. Auscultation of the chest reveals increased wheezes antero-ventrally. The heifer has a soft productive cough. The ruminal contractions are normal, occurring once per minute.

Routine haematological examination reveals a total red blood cell count of 4.1×10^{12}/L (4.1×10^6/µL) (normal range $5-9 \times 10^{12}$/L, $5-9 \times 10^6$/µL), leucocytes 12.4×10^9/L (12.4×10^3/µL) (normal range $4-10 \times 10^9$/L, $4-10 \times 10^3$/µL) with 65% neutrophils. Serum albumin and globulin concentrations are 24.8 g/L (2.48 g/dL) (normal range 30–40 g/L, 3–4 g/dL) and 61.3 g/L (6.13 g/dL) (normal range 35–45 g/L, 3.5–4.5 g/dL) respectively.
i. Which conditions would you consider? (Most likely first.)
ii. Comment upon the haematological and serum protein results.
iii. How could you confirm your provisional diagnosis?
iv. What treatment would you recommend?
v. What is the prognosis for this heifer?

16 A 4-day-old bull calf has been unable to bear weight on the right fore leg (16) since an assisted delivery in anterior presentation using a calving aid. The rectal temperature is 38.5°C (101.3°F). There is thickening of the umbilical stump. There is a loss of muscle tone and markedly reduced reflexes in the right foreleg but the left foreleg is normal. Normal reflexes are present in the pelvic limbs.
i. What conditions would you consider? (Most likely first.)
ii. What treatment(s) would you administer?
iii. What is the prognosis for this calf?

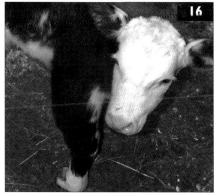

15 i. The most likely conditions to consider include: chronic suppurative pulmonary disease; liver abscessation/hepatocaval thrombosis; endocarditis; parasitic bronchitis; left-displaced abomasum (secondary to another disease process).

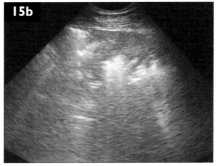

ii. Routine haematological examination reveals a mild anaemia consistent with chronic inflammatory focus. There is a slight leucocytosis resulting from a marginal neutrophilia. The changes in the serum albumin and globulin concentrations are consistent with chronic severe antigenic stimulation (e.g. bacterial infection).

iii. Auscultation of the chest is unreliable, and diagnosis of chronic suppurative pulmonary disease necessitates real-time B-mode ultrasonographic examination of the chest with a 5 MHz sector scanner, although linear array scanners can be used. The bright linear echo formed by normal visceral pleura at a depth of 2.5–3 cm from the probe head is present in the dorsal lung field but is replaced ventrally (10 cm above the point of the elbow; fifth and sixth intercostal spaces) by columnar hypoechoic areas extending up to 4–8 cm into the lung parenchyma (15b); this is consistent with localized (lobular) consolidation/cellular infiltration/abscess formation.

iv. *Arcanobacterium pyogenes* is most commonly isolated from such cases. The most effective treatment is 44,000 IU/kg procaine penicillin administered intramuscularly daily for 6 weeks.

v. The response rate for chronic suppurative pulmonary disease disease is about 50% depending upon severity (i.e. the extent of pathology determined ultrasonographically).

16 i. The most likely conditions to consider include: brachial plexus avulsion/radial nerve paralysis involving the right foreleg; septic arthritis of right foreleg joint (it may prove difficult to detect effusion/early infection in the shoulder/elbow joints); spinal cord trauma; congenital sarcocystosis.

ii. The calf was treated with intravenous flunixin. Procaine penicillin was injected intramuscularly daily for the next 5 days for the omphalophlebitis lesion. The calf was assisted to its feet and given basic physiotherapy every 4 hr. Splinting the distal limb should be considered if there is flexural contraction of the fetlock joint.

iii. The prognosis for such cases is very difficult to predict. This calf slowly improved over the next 2 weeks.

17 Figure **17a** shows a standing left laporotomy in a cow.

i. Identify the viscus and comment upon the incision site. Any further comments?

ii. What suture material and suture pattern would you use for closure?

iii. What else would you do before closing the abdominal incision?

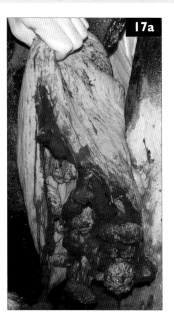

18 A 4-day-old bull calf from a beef herd is very dull and has been unwilling to suck for the past 36 hr. The calf appeared normal for the first 2 days and was observed to suck colostrum within the first 2 hr. The rectal temperature is 38.2°C (100.8°F). The calf is very depressed and weak but able to stand when assisted to do so. The calf is markedly dehydrated with sunken eyes and an extended skin tent beyond 5

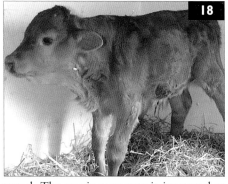

s. The mucous membranes appear congested. The respiratory rate is increased at 40 breaths per minute. The abdomen is markedly distended with fluid sounds audible on succusion. There is no evidence of diarrhoea and there are no faeces on the thermometer. There is thickening of the umbilical stump. The carcass lymph nodes are not enlarged.

i. What conditions would you consider? (Most likely first.)

ii. How could you confirm your diagnosis?

iii. What is the prognosis for this calf?

iv. What treatment(s) would you administer?

17, 18: Answers

17 i. This is the uterus. A straight incision has been made on the greater curvature; there are no tears. No drape has been used and the surgeon is not gloved/gowned. There is no placenta attached to caruncles: the calf was dead and the placenta was removed with the calf.

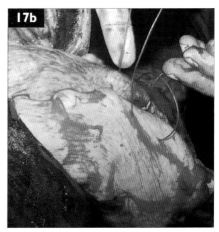

ii. The uterus should be closed with 7 metric chromic catgut in a single layer Connell pattern (inversion suture) (17b). Some surgeons recommend two suture layers but this approach is not necessary nor is it often possible due to the contracting uterus.

iii. The uterus is swabbed and all blood removed to reduce the risk of adhesions. The uterine wound is flushed with 1 L of sterile saline to remove all remains of blood clots. Any large blood clots can be scooped from the abdominal cavity. Intrauterine antibiotics are rarely used. Intra-abdominal antibiotics are used but with little convincing evidence for their efficacy.

18 i. The most likely conditions to consider include: atresia coli; omphalophlebitis and associated peritonitis; enterotoxigenic *Escherichia coli*; septicaemia; ruptured bladder with uroperitoneum; early meningoencephalitis; acidosis (but there is no evidence of diarrhoea).

ii. The diagnosis of atresia coli is based upon the clinical findings, particularly absence of any faeces by 4 days old. Transabdominal ultrasonography can investigate the umbilicus and guide abdominocentesis if excess accumulations of peritoneal fluid are identified.

iii. The prognosis for atresia coli cases is hopeless and calves should be euthanased once the diagnosis has been established.

iv. The calf was treated symptomatically with 5 L of isotonic saline over 6–8 hr, and intravenous trimethoprim/sulphonamide and flunixin meglumine. The calf's hydration status was much improved 6 hr later. The calf appeared much brighter but the abdomen was even more distended with fluid sounds on succusion. No faeces were passed in the 12 hr after first examination and the calf was euthanased for welfare reasons. Atresia coli was confirmed at postmortem examination.

19 In late summer a beef farmer complains that an autumn-calving cow grazing poor hill pasture before calving is 'going stiff'. The cow is isolated from the group and is dull and depressed (19). The cow has a gaunt appearance and is reluctant to walk. The rectal temperature is 40.0°C (104.0°F). The mucous membranes are congested. Rumen contractions are reduced. The respiratory rate is raised to 40 breaths

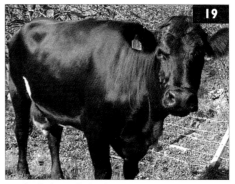

per minute. There is obvious distension of all four fetlock joints and both hock joints. The cow is not due to calve for 4 weeks, but the udder is swollen especially the right fore quarter. The right fore teat is very swollen and oedematous with flies clustered at the teat orifice.
i. What conditions would you consider? (Most likely first.)
ii. What is the cause?
iii. What treatments would you administer?
iv. What control measures would you recommend?

20 In late summer a group of 20 yearling beef heifers presents with poor growth and diarrhoea (20). Frequent nonproductive coughing after slight exertion has been heard over the past week. The heifers are set-stocked at three animals per hectare on permanent pasture. Clinical examination reveals normal rectal temperatures, absence of either ocular or nasal discharges, and occasional crackles audible on auscultation of the chest.

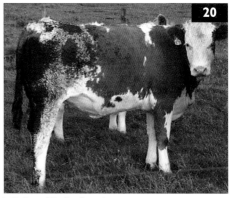

i. What conditions would you consider? (Most likely first.)
ii. What further tests could be undertaken?
iii. What treatment(s) should be administered?
iv. Could this problem(s) be prevented next year?

19, 20: Answers

19 i. The most likely conditions to consider include: summer mastitis; bacterial endocarditis; other chronic bacterial infections; redwater (babesiosis).
ii. Primary invasion of the mammary gland, with either the anaerobic organism *Peptococcus indolicus* or *Streptococcus dysgalactiae*, is followed by *Arcanobacterium pyogenes* infection to cause summer mastitis. There is circumstantial evidence only to link the sheep headfly *Hydrotaea irritans* with disease.
iii. The right fore quarter will not recover normal lactogenesis. Intramammary antibiotic infusion is ineffective due to the chronicity/extent of the infection although parenteral antibiotics, typically penicillin, are administered. Frequent stripping of the affected quarter every 2–4 hr is necessary to remove toxins and cellular debris but is not a simple procedure because of the painful oedematous teat. Lancing the teat in the vertical plane, thereby reducing the risk of haemorrhage associated with teat amputation, to facilitate drainage often produces disappointing results. NSAIDs, such as flunixin meglumine or ketoprofen, provide pain relief and stimulate appetite.
iv. Dry cow therapy/teat sealants remain the most effective means of preventing summer mastitis. Fly repellants, whether in the form of pour-on, spray-on or impregnated ear tag, provide useful protection against nuisance flies. Accessory teats should be removed before the animal is 6 weeks old.

20 i. The most likely conditions to consider include: lungworm; type I ostertagiasis; respiratory viral infections, including parainfluenza-3 and BRSV; poor pasture management; copper deficiency; BVD/MD infection (persistently infected animal in naïve group).
ii. Laboratory faecal examination (Baermann technique) will reveal patent parasitic infestations only. The modified McMaster technique for strongyle eggs can be used, either counting four to six individual samples or pooling samples together. Examination reveals *Dictyocaulus viviparus* L3 in three of six samples and a mean of 1,200 *Ostertagia ostertagi* eggs. Low serum copper concentrations samples from four to six calves would indicate depletion of liver copper reserves; normal values are recorded in this investigation.
iii. Treatment with an avermectin anthelmintic effects a good response (cessation of coughing and diarrhoea over the next few days) and provides protection against reinfestation for the remainder of the summer grazing period (cattle housed early autumn). Alternatively, the heifers could be treated with levamisiole followed by a group 1 benzimidazole anthelmintic (effective against hypobiotic larvae) administered at housing as the cheaper option.
iv. Where there is a known risk, lungworm is best prevented by vaccination 2 and 6 weeks before exposure. PGE control requires strategic anthelmintic treatment, including intraruminal pulse-release boluses (benzimidazole every 3 weeks), ivermectin injection 3, 8, and 13 weeks after turnout, doramectin injection at turnout and 8 weeks later, or doramectin slow-release injection at turnout.

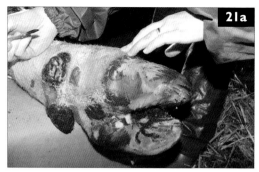

21 A 900 kg Limousin bull presents with severe lameness (9/10) of the right pelvic limb with marked muscle atrophy over the hip region. There is marked swelling of the bulb of the heel with loss of hair and thinning of the skin extending proximally to an area just below the accessory digits (21a). The distal limb is oedematous and pits under pressure. There is no widening of the interdigital space. Careful foot paring fails to reveal any hoof lesion.
i. What analgesia would you administer?
ii. What action would you take?

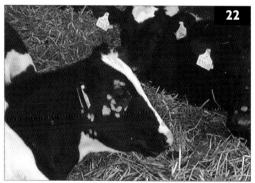

22 A group of 40 housed 4–6-month-old Friesian heifer calves is presented with numerous 2–6 cm diameter skin lesions distributed over the whole body but especially the head and neck (22). The lesions are superficial, dry, white, scaly, and nonpruritic. The affected skin is not thickened.
i. What conditions would you consider? (Most likely first.)
ii. Which further tests could be undertaken?
iii. What actions/treatments would you recommend?
iv. Are there any special concerns?

21 i. The bull should be sedated, e.g. with xylazine. Analgesia may be achieved by intravenous injection of lidocaine; a NSAID may also be used to provide analgesia. In this case, the bull is aggressive but is safely restrained in a bull crate with the leg hoisted. The bull has been lightly sedated with 45 mg xylazine (0.05 mg/kg) injected intravenously to remain standing. The right

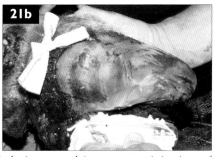

hindleg is hoisted and a tourniquet applied. Attempted intravenous injection of 30–40 mL of 2% lidocaine solution meets with forceful kicking (allodynia) and the crate is almost overturned. The bull is further sedated with 200 mg xylazine injected intramuscularly. At the same time 100 mL of 2% lidocaine are injected into the sacrococcygeal extradural space to paralyse both hindlegs for safety reasons and because it was not possible to find a superficial vein because of the distal limb oedema. Flunixin is injected intravenously when the bull is recumbent.

ii. A stab incision is made into the heel bulb abscess which releases pus and necrotic tissue. A blunt probe (index finger) is used to explore the extent of the lesion (10 cm to the coronary band), and further debride the lesion. A second stab incision is made at the distal margin of the lesion (bulb of the heel), and the abscess flushed repeatedly with a Penrose drain inserted (**21b**). A melolin dressing (or similar) is applied then cotton wool and a protective bandage applied using Elastoplast (or similar). A wooden block is applied to the sound claw (**21b**). Procaine penicillin is injected intramuscularly for 5 consecutive days. The dressing is changed after 4 days when the bull is 4/10 lame. The bull made a full recovery and is still in the herd 12 months later.

22 i. The most likely conditions to consider include: ringworm (*Trichophyton* spp. infection); lice (pediculosis); chorioptic mange; dermatophilosis; sarcoptic mange.

ii. Microscopic examination of hair/skin scrapings from the periphery of the lesions reveals fungal hyphae typical of *Trichophyton* spp. infection. Cultural examination can be undertaken on special media.

iii. Treatment includes topical natamycin application. In-feed griseofulvin medication for 10–14 days is available in some countries. There is the option of doing nothing, as lesions eventually regress with time (over 3–9 months) but in the interim the cattle do not look well and there is the risk of transmission to other livestock. Attentuated ringworm vaccine strain of *T. verrucosum* can be used in subsequent batches of calves.

iv. There is a zoonotic risk following contact with the calves or their environment.

Cow number	1	2	3	4	5	6	7	8	9	10
Milk yield L/day	34	34	32	33	41	31	26	26	27	32
BCS	3	2.5	2.5	2.5	3	2.5	3	2	2.5	2.5
3-OH butyrate										
mmol/L	**1.2**	**2.1**	**2.8**	**2.5**	**2.1**	**1.3**	**1**	**1.4**	**1.9**	**2.2**
(mg/dL)	**(12)**	**(21)**	**(28)**	**(25)**	**(21)**	**(13)**	**(10)**	**(14)**	**(19)**	**(22)**
Glucose mmol/L	**2.4**	**2.1**	**2.3**	**1.7**	**2.4**	**2.0**	3.1	**2.6**	3.0	3.2
(mg/dL)	**(43.2)**	**(37.8)**	**(41.4)**	**(30.6)**	**(43.2)**	**(36.0)**	(55.9)	**(46.9)**	(54.0)	(57.7)
NEFA mmol/L	0.3	0.4	**1.0**	**0.9**	0.2	0.3	0.2	0.2	0.2	0.2
BUN mmol/L	3.6	3.9	3.0	3.5	4.6	4.5	3.6	3.5	3.4	3.4
(mg/dL)	(10.1)	(10.9)	(8.4)	(9.8)	(12.9)	(12.6)	(10.1)	(9.8)	(9.5)	(9.5)
Albumin g/L	36	35	33	35	34	34	36	35	36	34
(g/dL)	(3.6)	(3.5)	(3.3)	(3.5)	(3.4)	(3.4)	(3.6)	(3.5)	(3.6)	(3.4)
Globulin g/L	44	46	39	41	45	43	42	42	46	41
(g/dL)	(4.4)	(4.6)	(3.9)	(4.1)	(4.5)	(4.3)	(4.2)	(4.2)	(4.6)	(4.1)

(Abnormal values in bold type.)

23 A farmer complains of poor fertility in his summer-calving dairy herd. The cows are fed 4–5 kg fresh weigh of concentrates twice daily in the milking parlour with access to grass silage (0.19 kg/kg DM, 10.5 MJ/kg/DM ME, and 156 g/kg crude protein) in ring feeders sited in the field. Computer analysis reveals an average ME requirement of 263 MJ/head/day with 92 MJ supplied from 8–10 kg of concentrates and maintenance plus 19 L of milk expected from forages (grazing plus silage). A metabolic profile of five early-lactation cows (1–5) and five mid-lactation cows (6–10), calved 3–6 weeks and 4 months respectively, is shown.
i. What are the major concerns from the cows' blood results?
ii. What are the potential causes of energy deficiency in this herd?
iii. What are the potential effects of energy deficiency on herd reproductive performance?
iv. What recommendations would you make?

24 Three of 120 fattening cattle have died suddenly over the last week. The cattle have been housed for 6 weeks and fed a high concentrate ration plus *ad libitum* potatoes and barley straw. Examination of blood smears has proved negative for anthrax.
i. What conditions would you consider? (Most likely first.)
ii. Which further tests could be undertaken?
iii. What control measures would you recommend?

23 i. The major concerns from the cows' blood results are the increased 3-OH butyrate and NEFA concentrations and decreased plasma glucose concentrations, indicating energy deficiency in both early-lactation and mid-lactation cows.
ii. A thorough review of feeding and husbandry practices is essential. Simple factors, such as the lack of grazing, buffer feed not available all day, and limited spaces at ring feeders, can severely restrict energy intake.
iii. The consequence of energy deficiency could include reduced fertility performance, manifest as a reduced submission rate (fewer cows presented for service by day 60 postpartum), cystic ovarian disease, poor oestrus expression, extended interval to first service, and lowered first service conception rate. More cows are presented for 'not seen bulling' by day 45 at routine veterinary visits.
iv. Recommendations could include providing buffer feed to all cows for only 2–3 hr per day prior to the afternoon milking. The protein status is satisfactory so extra energy can be provided by feeding an extra 2 kg/head/day of cereals (wheat, barley) to the lactating cows in the buffer feed. No more concentrates need to be fed in the milking parlour because levels are already too high, averaging 4.5 kg/feed. The bulk milk tank should be monitored (increased yield expected as well as fertility improvements), the herd resampled in 2 weeks, and the feeding strategy reassessed.

24 i. The most likely conditions to consider include: blackleg (clostridial myositis); choke; pasteurellosis; other septicaemic conditions including anthrax; electrocution from stray voltage; acidosis; thromboembolic meningoencephalitis.
ii. Further tests would include postmortem examination. Necropsy of the third dead animal reveals rapid autolysis and the musculature of the ventral neck is dry and dark purple with numerous gas pockets (**24**). These muscle groups contrast with normal adjacent muscles. The lungs are congested and oedematous.
iii. The farmer should be advised to vaccinate the remaining cattle against *Clostridium chauvoei* (blackleg) immediately. In this case all cattle were also injected with procaine penicillin at the time of vaccination to prevent the handling procedure from precipitating further cases. The second blackleg vaccine was given 2 weeks later. No further losses resulted in this group. Blackleg vaccine is cheap and a valuable insurance policy should losses from blackleg have previously occurred on the farm.

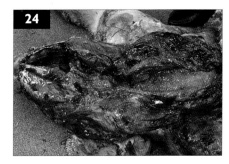

25 In early autumn you are called to a 4-year-old Limousin-cross-Friesian cow to assist delivery of a calf in posterior presentation. The cow is carrying her second calf sired by a Charolais bull. The cow is bright and alert and wandering around the calving box. The calf pelvic limbs are protruding from the vulva one hand's breadth short of the hock joints (25); the calf is alive.

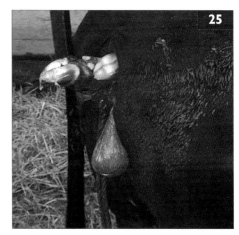

i. What guidelines can be applied to ascertain whether this calf can be delivered safely?
ii. What risks are associated with excessive traction in this situation?

26 A 15-month-old Limousin heifer presents with anorexia and is obtunded. The rectal temperature is 41.5°C (106.7°F). There is marked photophobia, blepharospasm, and corneal opacity. There are slight mucopurulent ocular and nasal discharges. The muzzle is markedly hyperaemic with sloughing of the overlying epithelium which bleeds readily on contact (26) There is increased salivation. There is a marked generalized peripheral lymphadenopathy. The heifer is hyperaesthesic to tactile stimuli,

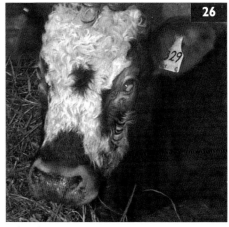

especially around the head. There are no skin lesions.
i. What conditions would you consider? (Most likely first.)
ii. What laboratory tests could be undertaken to confirm your provisional diagnosis?
iii. What treatment would you administer?
iv. What is the prognosis?
v. What control measures would you recommend?

25 i. The cow is haltered and the rope tied low down to a corner of a calving pen allowing approximately 1–1.5 m of rope. Examination reveals that the cervix is fully dilated and a hand can be extended over the calf's tail head and underneath both stifle joints.

The guideline for delivery of a calf in posterior presentation is that two strong people pulling on calving ropes should be able to extend the calf's hocks more than one hand's breadth beyond the cow's vulva (the calf's hindquarters are now fully within the pelvic inlet) within 10 minutes. Further traction will then deliver the calf safely (as happened in this case). With experience it is possible to apply greater traction than the forces described here and still achieve a successful resolution but there are occasional doubts when the calf becomes lodged. Is delivery of a live calf that subsequently dies a successful outcome?
ii. Risks associated with excessive traction include: (1) Calf – multiple rib fractures at the costochondral junction; rupture of the liver; prolonged delivery resulting in compression of umbilical vessels causing hypoxia/anoxia. (2) Dam – vaginal tear; rupture of middle uterine artery resulting in fatal haemorrhage. Nerve paralysis, such as obturator nerve paralysis, is much more common with calves delivered in anterior presentation.

26 i. The most likely conditions to consider include: malignant catarrhal fever; MD; thromboembolic meningoencephalitis; IBR encephalitis; bluetongue; bovine iritis (silage eye); rabies; foot and mouth disease.
ii. Malignant catarrhal fever virus can be identified in a peripheral blood sample by polymerase chain reaction.
iii. There are no specific treatments for malignant catarrhal fever and cattle should be carefully monitored and destroyed when it is clear they will not recover (this case). Successful treatment of malignant catarrhal fever with high doses of dexamethasone (1.0 mg/kg injected intravenously at first presentation) is rare. Antibiotic therapy may limit secondary bacterial involvement.
iv. The prognosis is very guarded with few confirmed recovered cases. Rarely, less severely affected cattle can survive but these cattle remain ill-thriven with a poor appetite. This heifer was euthanased immediately for welfare reasons.
v. Control of malignant catarrhal fever proves very difficult not least due to its sporadic occurrence. Malignant catarrhal fever is caused by a herpes virus transmitted from either sheep or deer. Separation of cattle from breeding ewes and deer is not always a practical option. The disease occurs very sporadically; one case every 5 years or so on mixed stock farms. Exceptionally, 10–20 cases of malignant catarrhal fever may occur on the same farm in the course of several months for no obvious reason.

27 An 11-month-old Limousin beef stirk is presented for veterinary examination after marked lameness of several months' duration. The stirk is 10/10 lame on the right forelimb with extensive muscle wastage and prominent spine of the right scapula. The rectal temperature is 39.2°C (102.6°F). There is extensive soft tissue swelling surrounding the right carpus. The carpal swelling is very firm, hot, and painful, with effusion of the radiocarpal joint. The right prescapular lymph node is ten times normal size. There are no other swollen joints.

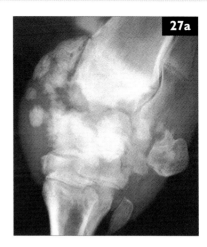

i. Describe the findings of the dorsopalmar lateromedial oblique radiograph (27a).
ii. What is the likely origin of this problem?
iii. What action should have been taken when the stirk was first noticed lame?

28 A yearling pedigree Charolais heifer presents with 8/10 lameness affecting the left hindleg having gone suddenly lame 3 months previously. The heifer has been penned on deep straw bedding. Initially the heifer had great difficulty rising but the severity of the lameness has reduced slightly although the animal spends much more time than normal lying down. There is extensive muscle

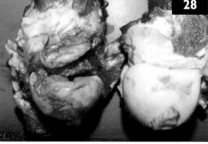

atrophy of the left gluteal muscle mass. Palpation of the left hindlimb fails to reveal any abnormality involving, or distal to, the left stifle joint. Lateral movement of the hindquarters produces a slight clunking sensation in the left hip region. There is no evidence of hip dislocation. The pelvis appears symmetrical. A diagnosis of femoral fracture through the proximal growth plate is based upon sudden onset with resultant chronic severe lameness originating above the stifle but not involving the pelvis. The heifer is euthanased for welfare reasons.

i. Describe the necropsy findings (28).
ii. What general advice would you offer to all clients regarding lameness to prevent similar cases of suffering?
iii. List those conditions causing severe lameness that fully recover after 3 months' 'rest'.

27 i. There is marked soft tissue swelling surrounding the carpus and marked ill defined, fluffy mineral opacities present surrounding the radiocarpal and intercarpal joints. The articular surface of the distal radius has been lost, there is patchy lysis of the distal radial epiphysis and mainly radial carpal bone, and widening of the radiocarpal joint. The distal intercarpal joint is widened and the carpometacarpal joint is ill

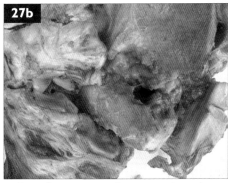

defined. The articular margins show osteophyte formation and some periosteal new bone formation is present on the proximal metacarpus, the carpal bones, and distal radius. The diagnosis is advanced chronic pancarpal arthritis and osteomyelitis, most likely septic (27b).

ii. The likely cause is a puncture wound penetrating the joint. Bacteraemia localized to one joint is unusual in growing cattle. There is no evidence of septic physitis extending into the joint.

iii. In view of the severity of the lameness, a serious condition should have been suspected and veterinary examination sought. The minimum treatment for a suspected joint infection would be parenteral antibiotic therapy and NSAIDs. Joint lavage is not a simple procedure in a 400 kg animal.

Veterinary examination is essential where the cause of severe lameness is not immediately obvious to the farmer for prognostic, economic, and welfare reasons. Euthanasia is indicated if the animal remains 10/10 lame after 1 week unless the cause has been accurately defined, correctly treated, and has a good prognosis. In this case it is clear that the animal has not received appropriate care.

28 i. There is a fracture through the proximal femoral growth plate.

ii. Veterinary examination is essential when there is sudden onset of severe lameness without obvious cause; it is also essential when the farmer believes he/she knows the cause(s), has given treatment(s), but there has been no improvement within 5 days. Where there is severe lameness and no response to veterinary treatment, euthanasia is indicated after no more than 1 week of onset of lameness.

iii. There are no conditions causing severe lameness that fully recover after 3 months' 'rest'.

29 You are presented with a 4-year-old Limousin bull with 2 days' history of right hindleg lameness. On assessment the bull is 8/10 lame and abducts the leg with the weight taken on the medial claw (29a shows the right hindfoot hoisted with the bull restrained in cattle stocks).
i. What conditions would you consider?
ii. What action would you take?

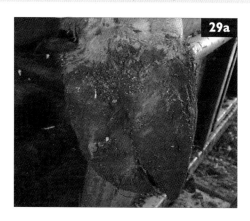

30 A Holstein cow, which calved 10 days ago, has no appetite and yielded only 4 L at her last milking. The cow is very dull and depressed, dehydrated with sunken eyes (30), and a skin tent extended to 5 s, consistent with >7% dehydration. Despite a reported poor appetite over the past 2 days, the abdomen looks distended. The rectal temperature is 38.4°C (101.1°F). The heart rate is 104 beats per minute and respiratory rate is 28 breaths per minute. Simultaneous percussion and auscultation reveal high-pitched pings over a 45 cm diameter area in the right sublumbar fossa, but the liver is not displaced from the right abdominal wall. Rectal examination fails to reveal any distended viscera and there are only scant faeces in the rectum. There is no melaena.
i. Comment upon the electrolyte concentrations listed.
ii. What action would you take?

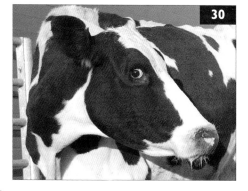

	Cow	Normal range
Chloride (mmol/L, mEq/L)	71	94–111
Potassium (mmol/L, mEq/L)	3.2	3.6–5.6
Sodium (mmol/L, mEq/L)	142	136–145
BUN (mmol/L)	24.5 (68.6 mg/dL)	2–6.6 (5.6–18.5 mg/dL)
GGT (IU/L)	364	20–46
AP (IU/L)	378	14–75

29 i. The most likely conditions to consider include: white line abscess in the lateral claw; penetration wound of the sole of the lateral claw; sole ulcer; laminitis.

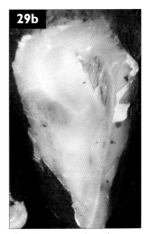

ii. The feet are overgrown and the lateral claw of the right hindleg is corkscrewed. The sole is pared and a black mark is detected in the white line of the abaxial wall more towards the heel region than the toe. Careful paring of the wall and sole following the black mark releases an abscess (29b; the toe is to the bottom of the image, the axial wall has not yet been pared). The abscess is pared out taking great care not to damage the corium. The foot is re-shaped. No bandage is necessary because there is no damage to the corium. Antibiotics are not necessary in this case because there is no tissue infection. The sole is thin as a consequence of paring out the abscess, the farmer is advised to house the bull on deep straw bedding for the next month while new horn growth takes place. Note the bruising of the sole at the site of a sole ulcer (29b). This is the classical site for a white line abscess in cattle: the lateral claw of the hindleg, and medial claw of the foreleg. The abscess is sited in the abaxial white line more towards the heel region than the toe because this is the site for greatest torsional forces when the foot contacts the ground, causing disruption of the white line and impaction of dirt and small stones leading to an abscess. The bull made an uneventful recovery. The bull's feet were trimmed using a bull crate 4 weeks after the first visit.

30 i. The clinical signs and electrolyte changes are compatible with pooling of chloride ions in the abomasum (hypochloraemia) and compensatory shift in potassium (hypokalaemia) in response to a metabolic alkalosis. These electrolyte disturbances are more severe than those normally encountered in cases of abomasal distension/right-sided displacement and may indicate early volvulus. The grossly elevated GGT is considered to result from biliary stasis as the cow has been inappetant for at least 2 days.

ii. The prognosis is guarded and surgery must be carefully considered because the heart rate above 100 beats per minute and serum chloride concentration <80 mmol/L (<80 mEq/L) indicate a poor prognosis.

Right flank laporotomy under paravertebral anaesthesia could be undertaken but should be preceded by the administration of intravenous flunixin meglumine and hypertonic saline (7.2%; 5 mL/kg in 5–7 minutes) followed by isotonic saline to stabilize the cow for standing surgery. Surgery may be ill advised in this case.

31 A 3-year-old beef cow presents with 2 months' history of weight loss and diarrhoea despite anthelmintic treatment by the farmer (**31a**). The heifer calved 3 months previously; the calf is not growing well. The rectal temperature is normal. No significant clinical signs are found except for profuse diarrhoea without blood or mucosal casts.

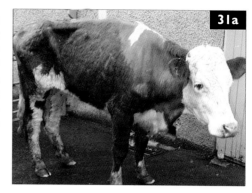

i. What conditions would you consider? (Most likely first.)
ii. Which further tests could be undertaken?
iii. What treatments would you recommend?
iv. What control measures could be adopted?

32 A beef farmer has approximately 200 fattening cattle in a slatted shed. Two stirks have lost varying lengths of the distal portion of the tail and the stumps have become septic with numerous discharging sinuses. The farmer did not worry unduly about this problem until one of the animals became lame with swollen joints and lost weight (**32;** the animal has

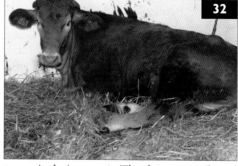

been moved from the slatted shed into an isolation pen). The farmer attributed this problem to laminitis caused by the high concentrate ration and slatted floor and did not pursue the problem any further until yesterday when this bullock was found dead. Postmortem examination confirmed the cause of death as bacterial endocarditis with the tail lesion as the probable primary septic focus.

The farmer has requested that the septic tail stump is removed from the other animal. The animal in question is bright and alert and in good bodily condition. The rectal temperature is normal (38.6°C (101.5°F)). The tail stump is septic with numerous discharging sinuses. There is no evidence of bacterial endocarditis but early lesions prove difficult to detect.

What would you do?

31, 32: Answers

31 i. The most likely conditions to consider include: Johne's disease (*Mycobacterium paratuberculosis*); chronic fasciolosis; persistent infection with BVD/ MD virus; chronic salmonellosis; type I or type II ostertigiasis; chronic bacterial infection leading to debility.

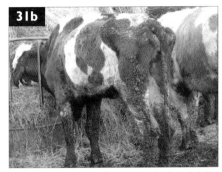

ii. The specificity of the ELISA test for Johne's disease is 97% but the sensitivity of this test is low until the latter stages of disease. If the clinical signs are suggestive of Johne's disease but the first sample proves negative, the animal should be quarantined and retested in 4–6 weeks. Culture of *Mycobacterium paratuberculosis* from faeces takes 4–6 weeks.

iii. The ELISA test for paratuberculosis is positive. There is no treatment for Johne's disease and all affected cattle and their progeny must be culled immediately to prevent further disease spread to young calves within the herd (**31b**).

iv. Control measures include improved biosecurity with the aim of a closed herd, free of disease. Where closed herd status is not possible, all breeding replacements, including bulls, should be purchased from a known source with no previous history of Johne's disease. Vaccination against Johne's disease prevents overt disease but is not an option for many beef farmers because replacement heifers are typically bought as either yearlings or in-calf heifers, and vaccination has to be undertaken within the first 2 weeks of life. Disadvantages of a vaccination policy include a granulomatous reaction at the injection site, cost, interference with the comparative intradermal tuberculin test, and trade/export restrictions.

32 Bacterial endocarditis can arise from a septic focus such as an infected tail, but not every septic wound will cause endocarditis.

The animal is restrained in cattle stocks. Caudal analgesia is effected by sacrococcygeal injection of 5 mL of 2% lidocaine solution (350–400 kg cattle). A tourniquet is applied as far proximally on the tail as possible. A V-shaped skin incision is made proximal to the infection on both the upper and lower surfaces. The tail is disarticulated using a scalpel blade at the first articulation above the level of the skin incision. The skin edges are sutured using nylon vertical mattress sutures. A pressure bandage is applied to the tail stump. It is not possible to evaluate the effectiveness of this surgery with respect to preventing future episodes of bacteraemia, and possible endocarditis.

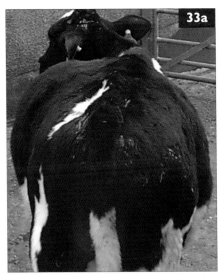

33 A 3-month-old 90 kg Holstein bull calf is presented with chronic bloat of 3 weeks' duration (33a). Although the bloat has been relieved twice daily for the past 4 days by stomach tube, the animal's condition is reported to be deteriorating. The calf's daily diet consists of 1 kg of a barley-based home-mix and hay *ad libitum*.

The calf appears alert and responsive. Gross distension of the left paralumbar fossa is noted. The calf's faeces are firm and notably fibrous, containing both undigested particles of hay and undigested barley. Rumen motility is depressed and no full contractions are heard. Palpation of the abdomen reveals dorsal left-sided gaseous distension. Below the gas layer, the ruminal contents feel firm. A stomach tube relieves the bloat completely.

i. What is your diagnosis?
ii. What treatment(s) would you recommend?

34 i. List the important diseases that your client could introduce into his beef farm by hiring a mature bull. (Most important first.)
ii. What control measures could you implement to reduce the risk of disease?

33 i. The most likely causes of eructation failure in calves include: inhibition of rumen motility caused by abnormal ruminal contents (i.e. indigestion); vagal lesions in the thorax resulting from respiratory disease (inflammation, abscess); vagal damage caused by abdominal inflammation; physical impairment of the cardia (polyps, inflammatory disease); painful abdominal conditions; abomasal displacement or distension.

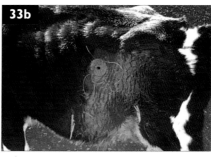

The findings of a firm, kneadable mass of ingesta occupying the ventral rumen along with firm, dry faeces with long undigested fibres indicate poor digestive function. A rumen sample reveals an alkaline rumen pH (>7), rapid sedimentation of particulate matter, sparse population of protozoa, and prolonged methylene blue reduction time of >15 minutes (normal <6 minutes), all indicative of simple inactivity of the ruminal microflora.

ii. The calf can be treated by administering 4 L of fresh ruminal transfaunate and 4 L of a commercial electrolyte solution via stomach tube, repeated 2 days later. In this case, the calf's condition progressively improved during the week following treatment. Bloat was relieved twice daily for 2 days and once the following day but was not required thereafter.

On occasion insertion of a rumen trochar may become necessary to relieve ruminal bloat while medical treatment is undertaken (33b).

34 i. The most important diseases to consider include: venereal disease, including *Campylobacter fetus venerealis*; BVD/MD persistently infected animal; Johne's disease; IBR; *Leptospira hardjo*; *Salmonella dublin* and other serotypes; tuberculosis; lungworm; fasciolosis; BRSV; lice.

ii. Control measures to reduce the risk of disease could include: (1) Premovement testing for tuberculosis. (2) During 1 month in strict quarantine following arrival collect the following samples: preputial sheath washing and culture for *Campylobacter fetus venerealis*; BVD/MD serology and antigen status; *Leptospira hardjo*, Johne's disease, BRSV, and IBR serology (vaccination status). (3) Treat for liver fluke and lungworm (where appropriate). (4) Treat for lice. (5) Ensure prompt veterinary examination for any illness.

35 A 6-month-old calf presents with a head tilt towards the right side and spontaneous horizontal nystagmus with the fast phase directed towards the left side. There is no circling behaviour. Ventral strabismus (eye drop) is present on the right side. There is drooping of the right upper eyelid and drooping of the right ear (35).

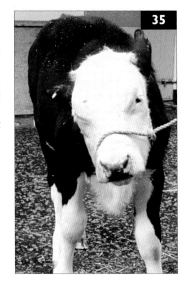

i. What conditions would you consider? (Most likely first.)
ii. What is the likely cause?
iii. What treatment would you administer?
iv. What is the prognosis for this case?

36 A Jersey cow that calved a week ago presents with 4 days' history of lethargy, poor appetite, and milk yield of 5 L/day. The cow had hypocalcaemia immediately after calving when she had been found cast on her back and extremely bloated. The cow responded well to intravenous calcium borogluconate. The cow now stands with a roached back stance with the neck extended and

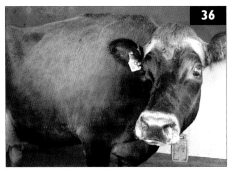

the head held lowered (36). The rectal temperature is elevated (39.4°C (102.9°F)). The ocular and oral mucous membranes are congested. There is a bilateral mucoid nasal discharge. The heart rate is 80 beats per minute. The respiratory rate is elevated to 44 breaths per minute with an obvious abdominal component. Auscultation of the chest reveals widespread crackles halfway down the chest wall on the right-hand side. Pinching over the withers elicits a painful expression. The ruminal contractions are reduced in strength and frequency.

i. What conditions would you consider? (Most likely first.)
ii. What tests would you undertake?
iii. What treatment would you recommend?

35 i. The most likely conditions to consider include: peripheral vestibular lesion; trauma to involve the middle ear/facial nerve; listeriosis.

ii. The vestibular system helps the animal maintain orientation in its environment, and the position of the eyes, trunk, and limbs with respect to movements and positioning of the head. Unilateral peripheral vestibular lesions are commonly associated with otitis media and ascending bacterial infection of the eustachian tube. There may be evidence of otitis externa and a purulent aural discharge in some cases but rupture of the tympanic membrane is not a common route of infection. *Pasteurella* spp., *Streptococcus* spp., and *Arcanobacterium* spp. have been isolated from infected lesions.

iii. A good treatment response is achieved with 5 consecutive days' treatment with procaine penicillin.

iv. The prognosis is very good in acute cases.

36 i. The most likely conditions to consider include: inhalation pneumonia; phlebitis/bacteraemia following calcium injection with a contaminated needle; chronic suppurative respiratory disease exacerbated after calving; pleurisy; hepatocaval thrombosis; endocarditis; peritonitis.

ii. Further tests would include routine haematology and serum protein analysis, and ultrasonography of the chest. There is a leucopenia (3.4×10^9/L (3.4×10^3/µL), normal range $4–10 \times 10^9$/L ($4–10 \times 10^3$/µL)), resulting from a marginal neutropenia (0.3×10^9/L, 0.3×10^3/µL) but a pronounced left shift with 22% immature neutrophils. There are marginal reductions in the serum albumin (29.9 g/L (2.99 g/dL), normal range >30 g/L (>3 g/dL)) and globulin concentrations (29.9 g/L (2.99 g/dL), normal range 35–50 g/L (3.5–5.0 g/dL)). The serum haptoglobin concentration is markedly elevated at 1.3 g/L (0.13 g/dL); normal <0.1 g/L (<0.01 g/dL).

A provisional diagnosis of inhalation/necrotizing pneumonia is based upon the clinical findings including pyrexia with pain on percussion supported by biochemical changes consistent with acute severe bacterial infection.

Real-time B-mode ultrasonographic examination of the chest with a 5 MHz sector scanner reveals separation of the pleurae ventrally with a 2 cm hypoechoic band and irregular 'columnar' hypoechoic areas extending up to 6 cm into the lung parenchyma consistent with pleurisy and severe lobular pneumonia, respectively.

iii. The cow was treated with marbofloxacin and flunixin meglumine injected intravenously. The cow was considerably worse 12 hr later and was euthanased for welfare reasons. A severe necrotizing pneumonia and associated pleurisy predominantly involving the right lung was evident at postmortem.

37 A 3-week-old Limousin-cross calf has been 9/10 lame for 3 days (37a). The right stifle joint is swollen, hot, and painful. There is an obvious joint effusion. The rectal temperature is 39.2°C (102.6°F). The right popliteal lymph node is not enlarged. No other joint lesions can be detected.

i. What would you do to investigate this problem further?
ii. How could effective analgesia be achieved?
iii. What action would you take?
iv. What is the likely prognosis?

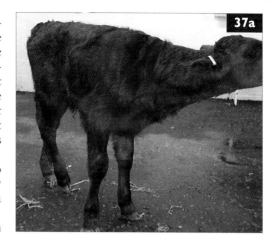

38 In early summer a 2-month-old beef calf presents as poorly grown with considerable faecal staining of the perineum, unlike other calves in the group. There is pale yellow, slightly mucoid diarrhoea which contains flecks of fresh blood. The calf is dull and appears gaunt with a tucked-up abdomen and a dry coat (38). There is frequent tenesmus with partial eversion of the rectum.

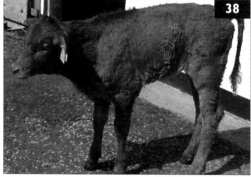

The calf is pyrexic (40.2°C (104.4°F)), with a slight mucopurulent nasal discharge. The submandibular and prescapular lymph nodes are enlarged.

i. What conditions would you consider? (Most likely first.)
ii. What tests would you undertake?
iii. What treatments would you administer?
iv. What is the prognosis?

37 i. The cause of the lameness could be investigated by arthrocentesis. The joint fluid sample is turbid with a protein concentration of 34.8 g/L (3.48 g/dL) (normal <3 g/L (<0.3 g/dL)) and a white cell concentration of 164×10^9/L (164×10^3/µL) comprised almost exclusively of neutrophils, confirming the diagnosis of septic arthritis.

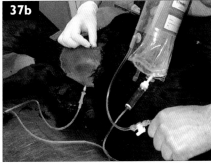

ii. Injectable general anaesthetic drugs, such as alphaxalone/alphadolone or propofol, may be considered prohibitively expensive and too short in duration of action. Intramuscular administration of 0.1 mg/kg of xylazine followed by intravenous administration of 2–3 mg/kg of ketamine is commonly used in practice. Incremental 2–3 mg/kg ketamine can be given to extend anaesthesia.

Effective analgesia after lumbosacral extradural injection of 3 mg/kg of 2% lidocaine solution allows a detailed and pain-free clinical examination of pelvic limb joint lesions and fractures and presents a cheap and readily available regime.

iii. The calf is injected with flunixin meglumine or other NSAID intravenously. The area over the right stifle joint is surgically prepared and two 16-gauge needles are inserted either side of the patellar ligament into fluid distensions of the joint. Once established in the joint, 1 L of Hartmann's solution is flushed through using a pressure pump device (37b) alternating the direction of flow through the needles. Florfenicol is commonly used for septic arthritis because *Salmonella* spp. are a common cause in older calves.

iv. The prognosis for septic arthritis is generally poor; however, this calf made good progress and was 3/10 lame when re-examined 2 days after joint lavage. It made an uneventful recovery. Prompt treatment is essential.

38 i. The most likely conditions to consider include: necrotic enteritis; coccidiosis; salmonellosis; intussusception; persistent infection with BVD/MD virus.

ii. The cause of necrotic enteritis has not been established. Where costs permit a lithium heparin blood sample should be submitted for BVD/MD status, and faecal samples submitted for both *Salmonella* culture and coccidial oocyst count with speciation of oocysts.

iii. Symptomatic treatments should be administered until test results are available; diclazuril for coccidiosis, and a 3-day course of florfenicol in the event of salmonellosis. A NSAID should be given daily for 3 days to control pain.

iv. The prognosis for necrotic enteritis is guarded.

39 You attend a beef heifer to assist delivery of a calf in anterior presentation with unilateral (right) shoulder flexion (leg back; 39). The calf is still alive despite the farmer applying considerable traction to the left leg using a calving jack.

i. How would you correct this malposture?

ii. What treatment(s) should be administered to the heifer?

iii. How should the calf be managed?

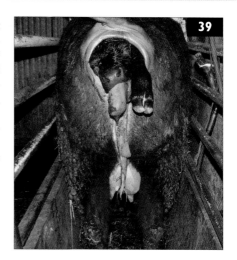

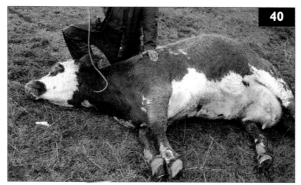

40 After a stormy autumn night you are called to attend a recumbent 10-year-old Simmental-cross-Friesian beef suckler cow that calved 36 hr ago (40). The cow is at pasture with a group of predominantly summer-calving cows which is receiving no supplementary feeding other than barley straw in a ring feeder. The cow was found by the farmer to be in lateral recumbency and 'thrashing wildly'. When you arrive the cow appears quiet but clinical examination precipitates seizure activity.

i. What conditions would you consider? (Most likely first.)

ii. What treatment would you administer immediately?

iii. What samples would you collect?

iv. What control measures could be adopted for the remainder of the herd?

39, 40: Answers

39 i. Correction of this malposture is best achieved with the cow standing in cattle stocks. Forceful straining during correction is prevented by injection of 5 mL of 2% lidocaine into the extradural space at the sacrococcygeal site. After 5 minutes the calf's head and left foreleg are well lubricated and slowly repelled until the calf's poll is level with the pelvic inlet. By first grasping the calf's right forearm then the mid-metacarpal region, the elbow and carpal joints are fully flexed which brings the calf's right foot towards the pelvic inlet. With the fetlock joint fully flexed, and the foot cupped in one's hand to protect the uterus, the foot is drawn forward into the pelvic canal extending the fetlock joint. Traction on the distal limb extends the elbow joint and the foot appears at the vulva where a calving rope is applied proximal to the fetlock joint.

The heifer should now be haltered and let out into a calving box. Steady traction of two people (veterinary surgeon and the farmer) pulling on the calving ropes applied to both legs will generally result in the heifer assuming lateral recumbency which aids delivery of the calf.

ii. Treatment should include a NSAID which should be given before commencing delivery of the calf; however, the considerable vulval oedema present (see 39) could also be treated with a single injection of dexamethasone. Antibiotics should be administered for 3 consecutive days because placental retention is likely after dystocia, and there is an increased risk of metritis.

iii. The umbilicus is immediately fully immersed in strong veterinary iodine, repeated 2 and 4 hr later. Two litres of colostrum should be administered by orogastric tube.

40 i. The most likely conditions to consider include: hypomagnesaemia; hypo-calcaemia; lead poisoning; bovine spongiform encephalopathy.

ii. While unlicensed for use in cattle, 6–8 mL of 20% pentobarbital solution injected intravenously controls seizure activity a great deal more effectively than either diazepam or xylazine. The cow is then haltered and 50 mL of 25% magnesium sulphate is added to a bottle of 400 mL of 40% calcium borogluconate solution and given by intravenous injection over 10 minutes. The remaining 350 mL of the bottle of 25% magnesium sulphate solution is given subcutaneously in two divided sites immediately behind the left shoulder. The cow was able to maintain sternal recumbency when pulled upright after all treatments had been administered and walked off to find its calf after a further 20 minutes.

iii. A serum sample for calcium and magnesium concentrations should be collected in case the cow does not respond to treatment.

iv. The farmer was advised to start feeding 2 kg per head per day of high-magnesium concentrates immediately. Good-quality barley straw should also be available *ad libitum*.

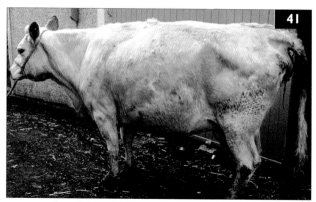

41 You are presented with a 6-year-old beef cow 5 days after a 'difficult breech calving' (posterior presentation with bilateral hip flexion) corrected by the farmer. The cow's rectal temperature is 38.4°C (101.1°F). The cow has a painful expression, a slightly arched back, and moves slowly (**41**). The udder contains little milk. The mucous membranes are congested and the cow is about 5–7% dehydrated. The heart rate is 96 beats per minute. The abdomen appears distended contrasting with the reduced appetite over the past 3 days. There are no rumen contractions heard over 3 minutes. There are no faeces in the rectum, only thick mucus. There is a reduced rectal sweep, restricting detailed examination of the abdomen.

i. What conditions would you consider?
ii. Which further tests could be undertaken?
iii. What actions/treatments would you recommend?

42 Calf hutches have become popular on dairy farms in the UK.
i. What advantages do calf hutches confer?
ii. Are there any disadvantages of this system?

41 i. The most likely conditions to consider include: diffuse septic peritonitis following uterine rupture; abdominal catastrophe – abomasal volvulus, intestinal torsion, proximal duodenal obstruction; traumatic reticulitis; metritis.

ii. Further tests include abdominocentesis and transabdominal ultrasonography. Abdominocentesis using an 18-gauge 38 mm needle at the ventral midline site immediately caudal to the xiphisternum yields a free flow of turbid straw-coloured fluid. The fluid has a protein concentration of 45 g/L (4.5 g/dL) and a white cell concentration of 1.8×10^9/L (1.8×10^3/μL) comprising 97% neutrophils, confirming the presence of peritonitis. Ultrasonography of the lower right flank revealed large volumes of fluid with numerous large fibrin tags.

iii. Diffuse septic peritonitis does not respond to antibiotic therapy. Peritoneal cavity lavage using large quantities of very dilute povidone–iodine solution has been reported to be successful in a limited number of early cases of peritonitis. However the extent of the fibrinous adhesions indicated that lavage would not be successful and the cow was euthanased for welfare reasons. The extent of the peritonitis was revealed at necropsy.

Rupture of the uterus is a risk when an unskilled person attempts to correct a breech calving. A low caudal extradural block is essential to prevent the cow straining during repulsion of the calf prior to extending the hindlegs. It must always be ensured that the umbilical cord does not become trapped around one of the hindlegs during such manipulation.

42 i. Calf husbandry using individual hutches enables the farmer to monitor the individual feed intake of all calves. There is no competition at feeding times which is important if feed is restricted. Rearing in individual hutches reduces infectious diseases due to lack of direct transmission of enteric and respiratory bacterial and viral pathogens. Individual penning prevents navel sucking behaviour. There is control of cryptosporidiosis and coccidiosis, however disease may occur when calves are later mixed into large groups unless husbandry standards are maintained.

ii. The major disadvantages of calves hutches is that they are expensive to install and maintain. It may be more time consuming with this system to feed calves, clean out, and disinfect pens between occupants. An alternative strategy is to move pens around a field after each occupant but hard road access is necessary in most situations. It is not possible to use automated milk delivery systems with calf hutches. There is exposure of calves/staff to adverse weather, and frozen water supplies in winter could be a problem. Access for routine procedures such as disbudding is time consuming. Individual penning removes the freedom to display normal behaviour, socialization, and interaction until moved into groups.

43 A 14-month-old Limousin heifer presents with 2 weeks' history of poor appetite and weight loss. Treatment with oxytetracycline by the farmer on two previous occasions had effected only slight improvement. The heifer had been purchased 3 months previously. The heifer is dull with a roached-back appearance. The rectal temperature is marginally elevated (39.2°C (102.6°F)). The

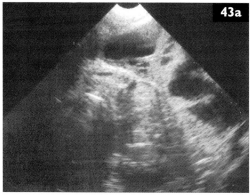

ocular and oral mucous membranes are congested. There is a mucopurulent nasal discharge. The heart rate is 72 beats per minute. The respiratory rate is elevated to 40 breaths per minute with a shallow abdominal component. The heifer has a soft cough. Auscultation of the chest reveals reduced breath sounds over the right chest.
i. Interpret the sonogram of the right chest (43a) obtained using a 5.0 MHz sector transducer connected to a real-time, B-mode ultrasound machine.
ii. What is the likely cause?
iii. What is the prognosis for this animal?

44 The laboratory values below were obtained from a 40 kg, weak, recumbent 10-day-old calf which has been scouring for the past 3 days. The calf has not responded to oral rehydration solution twice daily and parenteral antibiotics.
i. Comment on the clinically significant abnormalities.
ii. What treatment(s) would you administer?

Packed cell volume	0.31 L/L (0.24–0.36 L/L)
Total plasma protein	68.0 g/L (60–75 g/L)
	6.8 g/dL (6.0–7.5 g/dL)
Na	128 mmol/L (128–145 mmol/L)
K	7.2 mmol/L (3.6–5.6 mmol/L)
Cl	105 mmol/L (94–111 mmol/L)
Blood gas analysis:	
pH	6.9 (7.35–7.45)
pCO_2	46 mmHg
HCO_3	7 mmol/L (27–28 mmol/L)
Base deficit	20 mmol/L
(1 mmol/L is equivalent to 1 mEq/L)	

43 i. The parietal and visceral pleurae are separated by a 12 cm deep anechoic area spanned by many broad hyper-echoic bands, typical of a severe fibri-nous pleurisy.

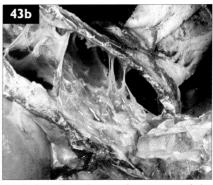

43b

ii. Such extensive fibrinous pleurisy (43b) is uncommon in bovine respir-atory disease in the UK and is probably related to earlier episodes of acute respiratory disease caused by *Haemo-philus somni* or *Mannheimia haemo-lytica*.

iii. The prognosis for such extensive pleurisy is hopeless due to the nature of the lesions causing physical impairment of lung function and inability to drain the chest. The animal should be destroyed for welfare reasons.

44 i. The calf does not appear dehydrated. The plasma protein concentration is consistent with passive antibody transfer (adequate colostrum ingestion). The sodium and chloride concentrations are normal. The very low bicarbonate con-centration and pH value indicate metabolic acidosis, probably as a consequence of diarrhoea and loss of bicarbonate/production of organic acids from secondary milk fermentation in the large intestine. The calf is hyperkalaemic following compensatory exchange of hydrogen ions for intracellular potassium ions. There may be a whole body depletion of potassium.

ii. Treatment must correct the acidosis. Total base deficit (or negative base excess) is calculated as:

$$\text{base deficit} \times \text{bicarbonate space (ECF)} \times \text{dehydrated calf weight}$$
$$= 20 \times (0.5) \times 40 = 400 \text{ mmol bicarbonate}$$
$$(\text{ECF: extracellular fluid volume})$$

32 g yielding 400 mmol of sodium bicarbonate can be added to 3 L of isotonic saline and administered over 3 hr with the first litre given over 20 minutes or so.

Follow-up fluids should comprise a high alkalinizing oral rehydration solution with 1 L offered by teat every 2 hr. Feeding should consist of alternate milk/oral rehydration solution administration rather than mixing these solutions in the same bottle. There is no justification for oral antibiotic administration but parenteral antibiotics are warranted if focal bacterial infection such as omphalophlebitis or polyarthritis is detected.

45 A 6-year-old Holstein cow presents with 6/10 lameness affecting the left hindleg. The onset of lameness was insidious but the severity has increased over the past 3 months and the cow spends much more time than normal lying down. The cow is bright and alert with a good appetite. There is normal anal and bladder tone. The tail is pulled toward the unaffected side caused by atrophy of muscles of the affected side (45a). Palpation of the left limb fails to reveal any abnormality involving, or distal to, the left stifle joint. There is a large firm swelling over the left hip. Lateral movement of the hindquarters produces a slight clunking sensation (crepitus) felt over the left hip region. Rectal examination reveals no pelvic abnormality.

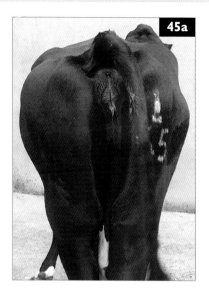

i. What conditions would you consider?
ii. How could you confirm your diagnosis?
iii. What action would you take?

46 Overnight, a 9-month-old (360 kg) Holstein bull presents with a very large swelling of the ventral abdomen, which extends from the scrotum to the xiphisternum and pits under digital pressure (46). The bull appears uncomfortable and often adopts a wide stance with the hindlimbs placed further back than normal. He has a normal appetite. The rectal temperature is normal (38.5°C (101.3°F)). A normal flow of

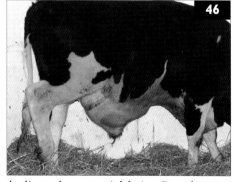

urine is voided. There are numerous calculi on the preputial hairs. Rectal examination reveals no abnormality. There is a skin break across the middle of the swelling.

i. What conditions would you consider?
ii. What further clinical examinations should be undertaken?
iii. How would you correct this problem?
iv. What control measures could be adopted?

45 i. The most likely conditions to consider include: severe hip arthritis with
fibrosis/oedema of the joint capsule; deep-
seated abscess/cellulitis post injection;
dislocated hip; septic hip joint; femoral
fracture involving the greater trochanter;
pelvic fracture involving the acetabulum.
There is no evidence of hip dislocation
(upward and cranial displacement). The
pelvis appears symmetrical. A diagnosis of

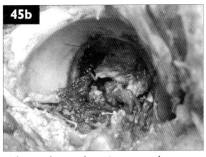

hip arthritis is based upon insidious onset with resultant chronic severe lameness
originating above the stifle but not involving the pelvis. The clunk could be caused
by slight movement across a fracture site or, more likely, increased joint laxity and
greater movement of the femoral head within the acetabulum. However, joint
movements are restricted by the surrounding tissue reaction and muscle mass.
ii. Osteoarthritis is very difficult to diagnose. The overlying muscle masses and
periarticular reaction would present considerable problems with interpretation of
ultrasound images of the hip joint but such examination would identify deep-seated
abscess(es). Radiography necessitates dorsal recumbency and either deep sedation or
general anaesthesia and a powerful machine for cattle >500 kg. Casting the cow,
positioning for, and recovery from radiography may exacerbate any existing lesion.
iii. The cow must be euthanased immediately even without radiographic confirmation of the suspected hip arthritis. Necropsy revealed extensive fibrous tissue
reaction surrounding the joint with almost complete erosion of articular surfaces
which were separated by an organized blood clot which may explain the 'slight
clunk' only (45b).

46 i. The most likely conditions to consider include: ruptured penis and massive
haematoma formation; cellulitis from puncture wound of the ventral abdomen wall;
infectious balanoposthitis; partial obstructive urolithiasis with urethral rupture.
ii. The BUN concentration is only marginally elevated at 7.8 mmol/L (21.8 mg/dL)
(normal range 2–6 mmol/L, 5.6–16.8 mg/dL). Ultrasound examination may aid
diagnosis, but it may prove difficult to differentiate recent haemorrhage from
subcutaneous urine accumulation. A fine-needle aspirate can be collected under
strict asepsis. Urine can be differentiated from other body fluids by measuring
electrolyte and creatinine concentrations. The diagnosis is a penile haematoma.
iii. The massive haematoma formation will resolve over several months.
iv. Secure accommodation must be maintained. The farmer had found the bull
suspended halfway over a metal gate dividing two pens. The manure in the pens
had been allowed to become too deep and the gate was now too low.

47 In mid-autumn you attend a group of 64 housed beef cattle aged 9–12 months, purchased from numerous markets over the previous 3 weeks. Frequent coughing has been heard in the group over the past week. The farmer has selected two inappetant animals with purulent ocular and nasal discharges (47) for veterinary examination. Clinical examination reveals pyrexia (40.8 and 41.1°C (105.4 and 106.0°F), respectively). The respiratory rate is increased and auscultation of the chest

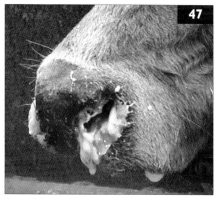

reveals crackles but these sounds are transferred from the upper respiratory tract. Visual inspection of the remainder of the group reveals a number of cattle with mucopurulent ocular and nasal discharges and tachypnoea. Six animals are selected and examined, all of which have a rectal temperature >40.5°C (104.9°F).
i. What conditions would you consider? (Most likely first.)
ii. How would you confirm your diagnosis?
iii. What treatment (s) would you recommend?
iv. What control measures could be adopted for future years?

48 In mid-autumn a farmer reports a single beef cow which is febrile (40.0°C (104.0°F)) and appears stiff and very reluctant to move due to swelling of the coronary band at the top of the hooves. There is a serous to mucopurulent nasal discharge and there are erosions on the muzzle with sloughing of the mucosa (48). There is lacrimation but no obvious eye lesions.
i. What conditions would you consider?
ii. What action would you take?
iii. How is the provisional diagnosis confirmed?
iv. What control measures could be considered?

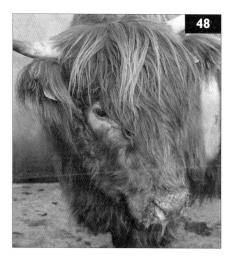

47 i. The most likely conditions to consider include: IBR; pasteurellosis; blue-tongue; BRSV infection.
ii. Many animals in the group are febrile suggesting a viral aetiology. Ocular swabs (vigorous action to obtain cellular material) for FAT for IBR are taken from four to six febrile cattle with a serous discharge. If the swabs cannot be delivered to the laboratory that day, they should be smeared on to glass slides and air-dried. Results of FAT should be available within hours. Paired serology would involve 2 weeks' delay.
iii. The farmer is advised to vaccinate all cattle immediately with an intranasal IBR vaccine. All sick cattle are treated with an intramuscular injection of procaine penicillin at 44,000 IU/kg for 3 consecutive days and then re-examined. No clinical advantage is gained by using one of the much more expensive antibiotics such as florfenicol or tulathromycin.
iv. Vaccination against IBR upon arrival on the farm is very effective and affords life-long protection. Animals should be quarantined for at least 2 weeks after arrival on the farm.

48 i. Single cases of bluetongue were first reported in the UK during August 2007. The most important differential diagnosis is foot and mouth disease, where the infection causes profuse salivation, erosions/ulcers in the mouth, lameness, and fever spread rapidly to affect all cattle on the premises within days. Other important differential diagnoses include IBR (group or herd) and malignant catarrhal fever (usually individual cattle). Bacterial endocarditis and chronic mastitis can cause fever and lameness with reluctance to walk but there are no head signs.
ii. Bluetongue is a notifiable disease in the UK and suspected cases must be reported immediately to the local Animal Health Office.
iii. Diagnosis is confirmed following virus isolation and/or seroconversion to bluetongue virus.
iv. Control of bluetongue is very difficult because of the large number of potential hosts and virus serotypes. While control is aimed at keeping susceptible animals away from the vector this is not always practical. Control of the *Culicoides* vector can be attempted with pour-on insecticides, but this is expensive and does not achieve total freedom from the midge. Killed vaccines are used extensively worldwide and were successfully used in the UK in 2008. Most modified live vaccines produce a viraemia in the vaccinated animal which affords the opportunity for further spread. Problems may arise with viral reassortment if viraemic animals are vaccinated with a modified live vaccine. The timing of vaccination will depend upon local factors, in particular the occurrence of high-risk periods.

49 In winter you are presented with a 9-month-old, 220 kg Blue-grey heifer with 3 days' history of anorexia and slight bloat. The heifer presents with a wide-based stance (49a), and walks reluctantly with a very stilted gait. The tail is held rigidly away from the rump. The heifer has an anxious expression with the ears erect and nostrils flared. The third eyelid is more evident than normal. There is constant drooling of saliva and it is not possible to open the heifer's mouth. The rectal temperature is normal. The heart rate is 94 beats per minute and respiratory rate of 24 breaths per minute. No rumen contractions are heard over 3 minutes.

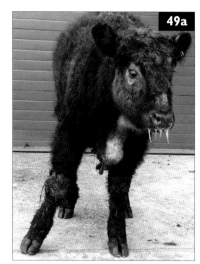

i. What conditions would you consider?
ii. What supportive therapy could be administered?
iii. What is the likely source of infection?

50 You are presented with a 2-week-old Holstein bull calf which the farmer reports has been unsteady on its legs since birth and appears unaware of its surroundings. The calf has a lowered head carriage, intention tremors, and a wide-based stance (50a). The calf is ataxic with hypermetria of all four legs but normal strength. The calf has no menace reflexes but normal pupillary light responses. No other cranial nerve deficits are detected.

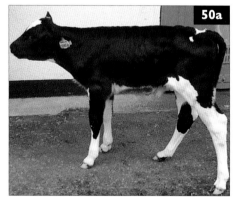

i. What area(s) of the brain could be involved?
ii. What causes would you consider?
iii. What other signs might you expect?

49 i. The most likely conditions to consider include: tetanus; trauma to the cervical vertebral column/spinal cord (C2–C6); lead poisoning; thromboembolic meningoencephalitis; bacterial meningoencephalitis following septicaemia.

ii. Symptomatic treatment includes high doses of procaine penicillin admin-

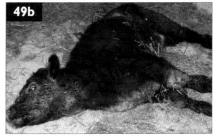

istered intravenously. The heifer is sedated with 20 mg acetylpromazine (0.1 mg/kg) every 8 hr. The heifer deteriorated overnight (49b) and was euthanased for welfare reasons. No further cases occurred in this group.

iii. This group of heifers was being fed poor-quality big bale silage and it is possible that soil contaminated with *C. tetani* and abnormal fermentation permitted bacterial proliferation and toxin production causing disease.

50 i. The clinical signs are suggestive of both a cerebellar lesion (wide-based stance, low head carriage, intention tremors, ataxia, dysmetria but normal strength) and cerebral lesion (altered mental state, lack of menace response).

ii. The calf has shown clinical signs since birth therefore a congenital rather than a developmental lesion would be suspected. This fact excludes cerebellar abiotrophy and infections such as meningoencephalitis and brain abscess(es).

The most likely conditions to consider include: hydranencephaly; cerebellar aplasia/hypoplasia; cervical spinal lesion; atlanto-occipital joint infection.

A diagnosis of hydranencephaly (50b at necropsy) was considered to be the most likely diagnosis. The possible involvement of BVD/MD virus infection during fetal development could not be examined until the calf is around 2 months old because of the presence of maternally derived antibody in the calf (unless the dam was a persistently infected BVD/MD animal herself and therefore seronegative). Congenital Akabane virus infection should also be considered in certain parts of the world.

iii. Other defects caused by BVD/MD virus include cataracts, skeletal deformities such as kyphoscoliosis, flexural deformities of the limbs, and brachygnathia.

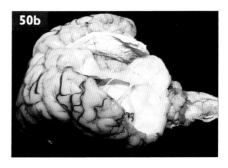

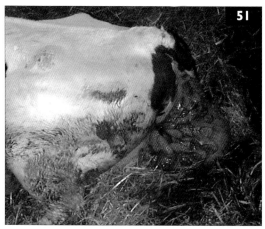

51 At 5 am you are presented with a recumbent 7-year-old Friesian cow which calved at some stage during the night and now has a uterine prolapse (51). The cow's head is averted against her chest and she is unable to gain her feet. There is moderate bloat.

i. How would you correct this problem?
ii. What treatments will you administer?

52 A six year-old Friesian cow has been unable to regain her feet since an assisted calving during which the calf became 'hip-locked' and was eventually delivered by the farmer using a calving aid. The farmer has since transported the cow out into a small field to provide a nonslip surface (52). The cow is in sternal recumbency, bright and alert, afebrile (38.5°C (101.3°F)), with normal mucous membranes, heart rate of 82 beats per minute, and a normal respiratory rate (20 breaths per minute). The cow has made a number of attempts to rise but 'her hindlegs go sideways'.

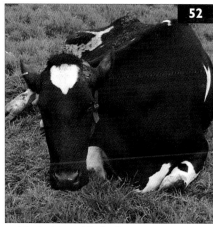

i. Which diseases/conditions would you consider? (Most likely first.)
ii. How would you manage this case?

51, 52: Answers

51 i. The uterus is replaced after sacrococcygeal extradural injection of 6 mL of 2% lidocaine. The cow is haltered and rolled on to her sternum and the pelvic limbs positioned behind with the hips fully extended and the weight of the cow's hindquarters taken on her stifle joints. The fetal membranes are carefully detached from the caruncles if possible. The prolapsed uterus is cleaned in warm dilute povidone–iodine solution and any gross contamination removed. The uterus is then held at the level of the vulva and replaced, starting at the cervical end. At first there seems to be little progress but eventually the uterine horn is replaced into the vagina and carefully returned to its normal 'comma-shaped' position. The pelvic limbs are returned to their normal flexed position. The prolapsed tissues can be retained using a Buhner suture of 5 mm umbilical tape but this is unnecessary when the prolapse is associated with hypocalcaemia.
ii. Treatment includes the intravenous administration of 400 mL of 40% calcium borogluconate given slowly over 10 minutes with the heart rate monitored throughout infusion. Oxytocin (40 IU) is given intramuscularly. The cow is treated with parenteral oxytetracycline for 3 consecutive days to prevent metritis. The cow was checked 21 days after calving as part of the herd fertility control programme and treated with prostaglandin F2 alpha for chronic endometritis.

52 i. The most likely conditions to consider include: trauma at parturition resulting in obturator nerve paralysis; hypocalcaemia; fractured pelvis/femur; coliform mastitis; other infectious conditions causing toxaemia/endotoxaemia.

No abnormalities of the posterior reproductive tract/uterus are detected on vaginal examination. No abnormalities of the pelvis could be detected on rectal examination or palpation. No long bone fractures could be detected. A diagnosis of obturator nerve paralysis was based upon the lack of another reason for recumbency, and history of 'doing the splits' after an assisted calving. Since the obturator nerve provides sensory innervation to the medial thigh, skin test responses in this region could be useful but access may present problems.
ii. Predicting the duration of recumbency proves very difficult and the cow could regain her feet within days, after 3 weeks, or may never rise. The cow's pelvic limbs can be hobbled just above the fetlock joints but they must be checked regularly for skin abrasions. The udder should be checked twice daily for mastitis. Food and fresh water must always be available and within reach. The cow must be turned regularly unless she is moving around the field herself. There is no convincing published evidence for the use of hoists, inflatable cushions, and webbing nets. Bagshaw hoists (the animal is hoisted by a device spanning the wings of the ilium) must never be used. Good results are claimed for flotation tanks but such apparatus is rarely seen on farms. The level of care on busy commercial dairy farms is rarely adequate and recumbent cows are usually killed for welfare reasons after a week or so.

53 i. Identify this instrument (53) and its purpose.
ii. What advantages, if any, does it confer over other techniques?
iii. Are there any disadvantages of this technique?

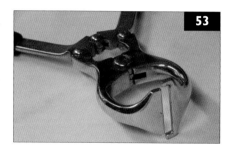

	I	2	3	4	5	6	Normal
Milk yield L/day	46	39	44	48	46	48	
BCS	3	3	2	1.5	3	1.5	
3-OH butyrate mmol/L	**1.2**	**1.1**	**1.8**	**4.5**	0.9	0.8	<0.8
(mg/dL)	**(12)**	**(11)**	**(18)**	**(45)**	(9)	(8)	(<8)
Glucose mmol/L	3.3	3.7	**2.6**	**1.8**	3.4	3.3	>3.0
(mg/dL)	(59.5)	(66.7)	**(46.9)**	**(32.4)**	(61.3)	(59.5)	(>54.0)
NEFA (mmol/L)	0.3	0.4	0.3	**0.9**	0.2	0.3	<0.7
BUN mmol/L	3.6	3.9	3.0	3.5	4.6	4.5	2.2–6.6
(mg/dL)	(10.1)	(10.9)	(8.4)	(9.8)	(12.9)	(12.6)	(6.2–18.5)
Albumin g/L	36	35	33	35	34	34	30–40
(g/dL)	(3.6)	(3.5)	(3.3)	(3.5)	(3.4)	(3.4)	(3.0–4.0)
Globulin g/L	44	46	39	41	45	43	35–45
(g/dL)	(4.4)	(4.6)	(3.9)	(4.1)	(4.5)	(4.3)	(3.5–4.5)
(Abnormal values in bold type)							

54 A farmer complains that his high-yielding cows are not meeting expected peak milk yields, with a low milk protein concentration (average 3.05%; target >3.4%). The cows are fed 40 kg grass silage (0.23 kg/kg DM, 10.6 MJ/kg/DM ME, and 135 g/kg crude protein) and 14 kg fresh weigh of concentrates in a total mixed ration. Computer analysis reveals an average ME requirement of 283 MJ/head/day with 162 MJ supplied from concentrates and maintenance plus 10 L of milk expected from forage. A metabolic profile of six cows (plasma samples), calved 3–6 weeks, is shown. The average BCS in early lactation is 2.3 compared to 3.4 in the dry group (scale 1–5).
i. What is the likely cause of the low milk protein concentration?
ii. What are the major concerns from the cows' blood results?
iii. What are the potential causes of energy deficiency in this herd?
iv. What are the potential consequences of energy deficiency?

53 i. This instrument is a Burdizzo clamp for bloodless castration.
ii. Evidence produced in calf and lamb castration studies show the acute phase pain-induced distress caused by Burdizzo clamp is significantly less than surgery because the crushing process destroys the nerve fibres. There is no risk of ascending infection unlike surgical wounds. Tetanus is very occasionally reported following infection of surgical castration wounds.
iii. While there are welfare benefits from use of the Burdizzo clamp, there are also some risks. Care must be taken to crush both spermatic cords correctly because failed castration would leave a fertile male and the potential for unwanted pregnancies in any sexually mature heifers in the group (occasionally encountered in beef calves). Ideally, calves should be checked 2–4 weeks after Burdizzo castration for testicular atrophy. Surgical castration in cattle where the Burdizzo procedure has not been performed correctly proves very difficult because of adhesions between the vaginal tunics.

On occasion farmers have mistakenly crushed the penis/urethra resulting in urethral obstruction and eventual death of the calf. The Burdizzo technique is not simple in cattle with a short scrotum or when there is a lot of fat deposited within the scrotum in over-conditioned beef calves.

54 i. The likely cause of the low milk protein concentration is energy deficiency over several months.
ii. Increased 3-OH butyrate and NEFA concentrations and decreased plasma glucose concentrations indicate energy deficiency in the early lactation cows. This is supported by the loss of one unit of condition score during early lactation (target 0.5 unit).
iii. There are many potential causes of energy deficiency and care must be taken not to over-interpret blood results without a thorough review of feeding and husbandry practices. Simple factors, such as the feed being available all day, easy access for all cows, sufficient comfortable cubicles, can all affect feed intake, rumination, cow comfort, and ultimately energy status. If there are no obvious problems with feed delivery, feeding an extra 2 kg/head/day of cereals (wheat, barley) to the early lactation group should be considered.
iv. The consequence of energy deficiency could include clinical acetonaemia (cow 4 is at risk). In the longer term, excessive loss of body condition and reduced fertility performance manifest as a reduced submission rate (fewer cows presented for service by day 60 postpartum), poor oestrus expression, extended interval to first service, and lowered first service conception rate. More cows are presented for 'not seen bulling' by day 45 or so.

55 You are instructed to dehorn a group of 6–7-month-old spring-born beef calves (220–270 kg). The farmer reports that the spring-born calves could not be dehorned until the end of the fly season, and in this case not until housing in late autumn (55a).

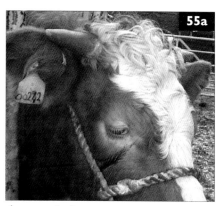

i. What dehorning practices would you use routinely?
ii. What method would you use in this instance?
iii. How do you know your analgesia has been effective?
iv. Do you agree with your client's husbandry practice?

56 A 7-year-old dairy cow presents with a 4 week history of continuous salivation, and frequent reflux of 20–30 mL of saliva/rumen liquor from the nostrils and mouth followed immediately by a moist cough. The appetite is poor but there is slight abdominal distension and loss of condition (now BCS 1.5; scale 1–5). The cow can swallow small quantities of masticated food but the food bolus is more obvious than normal because the oesophagus appears dis-

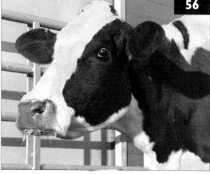

tended. The cow has not been noted ruminating. The cow has a roached-back appearance and an anxious expression; refluxed fluid is apparent around the nostrils and on the muzzle (56). The rectal temperature is normal. The pulse rate is 52 beats per minute. There is obvious jugular distension. The submandibular and retropharyngeal lymph nodes are two to three times larger than normal. The rate of rumen contractions is increased to approximately three to four cycles per minute (normal one cycle per 40 s or so) but the intensity of sounds is decreased. The faeces are soft and contain a high percentage of long fibre. The withers pinch test (Williams' test) is negative. A stomach tube releases only a small amount of gas.
i. What conditions would you consider? (Most likely first.)
ii. How would you confirm your diagnosis?
iii. What actions/treatments would you recommend?

55 i. It is preferable to disbud calves within the first month of life using a hot disbudding iron after subcornual nerve block with lidocaine rather than the scoop method, because cautery disables nociceptor transmission from the site and causes much less acute phase pain-induced distress.

ii. In older calves a subcornual lidocaine nerve block is used. The large blood vessels are twisted with artery forceps after removing the horns with

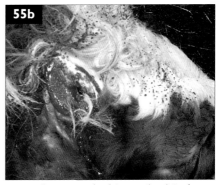

guillotine shears (55b), rather than cauterizing the wound; this method is faster and cautery often fails to stops arterial spurting. It may prove less painful if the wound edges are cauterized, destroying nerve endings, but the cauterized wound may take longer to heal and be more prone to secondary bacterial infection.

A NSAID should be given intravenously prior to dehorning. The addition of xylazine to the lidocaine solution used for subcornual block aids handling of fractious cattle (approximately 4 mL of 2% xylazine to 100 mL 2% lidocaine).

iii. Analgesia can be tested by lack of response to skin prick around the horn base more than 5 minutes after injection, and observation of ptosis (shown in 55a and b).

iv. There can be few genuine reasons why these calves were not disbudded within the first few weeks of life.

56 i. The most likely conditions to consider include: megaoesophagus resulting from mediastinal mass, e.g. a thymic lymphosarcoma or reticular abscess; pharyngeal/oesophageal hypomotility/paralysis; lesion at the cardia; vagus indigestion.

ii. A diagnosis of vagus indigestion (rumen hypermotility, bradycardia) does not explain the reflux of rumen liquor. Ultrasonographic examination of the anterior abdomen using a 5 MHz sector scanner failed to detect any abdominal abscess. Endoscopy revealed dorsal displacement of the soft palate and lack of propulsive motility along the whole length of the oesophagus. The flaccid oesophagus contained small pockets of rumen liquor. The cardia appeared normal with no obstruction or mass.

A diagnosis of pharyngeal/oesophageal hypomotility/paralysis was reached; the cause could not be determined.

iii. The prognosis in this cow was considered to be very poor due to the chronicity and loss of oesophageal function. The cow was slaughtered on the farm for welfare reasons. No postmortem results are available.

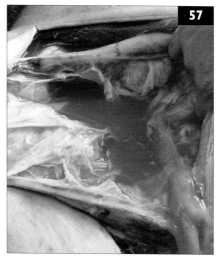

57 Necropsy of a 4-year-old beef cow 2 weeks after a 'difficult calving' (both calves presented simultaneously) corrected by the farmer reveals the image shown in 57. The cow had been normal for the first few days, but thereafter she had a poor appetite and both calves were reared artificially due to the cow's poor milk yield. The cow had received two courses of antibiotics (5 consecutive days' procaine penicillin, then two injections of florfenicol) but with little improvement. The cow had an arched back and moved slowly. The abdomen distension contrasted with the poor appetite.

i. Describe the findings in 57.

ii. Which further tests could have been undertaken on the farm had the cow been presented when first noticed ill?

iii. What actions/treatments could have been administered when the cow first became ill?

iv. What prevention measures would you recommend?

58 A 18-month-old Limousin-cross heifer presents with a drooped jaw, pro-truding tongue, and salivation. The heifer experiences considerable difficulty prehending and masticating food. The heifer is housed and this condition was not noted the previous day.

i. What conditions would you consider? (Most likely first.)

ii. Which further tests could be undertaken?

iii. What actions/treatments would you recommend?

iv. What is the probable cause?

57 i. There is an extensive fibrinous matrix with large volumes of turbid yellow (foul-smelling?) fluid released from the abdominal cavity, consistent with diffuse septic peritonitis.

ii. Abdominocentesis at the ventral midline immediately caudal to the xiphister-num is commonly used; an alternative site is on the right-hand side cranial to the udder. (The 'four quadrant' approach is rarely used in practice.) Septic peritonitis yields a turbid sample with a protein concentration >3 g/L (>0.3 g/dL); often >30 g/L (>3.0 g/dL) with increased white cell count and >95% neutrophils. In more advanced cases the needle point may be introduced into fibrin deposits yielding no sample and a misleading result. Ultrasound-guided centesis is helpful.

In peritonitis cases, ultrasonography initially reveals accumulation of inflammatory exudate with the appearance of fibrin tags after 24–48 hr.

iii. It is essential to establish a specific diagnosis because the outcome of peritoneal infection depends upon the origin of infection, involvement of adjacent organ(s), and the ability of the omentum to localize infection. Traumatic reticulitis and focal peritonitis respond reasonably well to antibiotic therapy if detected within 24 hr and the wire is recovered, while only a few fibrin tags constricting the small intestine (e.g. proximal duodenal obstruction) can cause severe disease and ultimately death. The diagnosis involves a careful clinical examination, assessment of heart rate, percussion/succussion, electrolyte deter-minations (chloride particularly), ultrasonography, and in some cases explorative right flank laporotomy.

iv. This scenario could have been prevented by veterinary assistance when the dystocia was first identified.

58 i. The most likely conditions to consider include: fracture of the left horizontal ramus of the mandible; wooden tongue (*Actinobacillus lignieresii* infection); osteomyelitis – lumpy jaw (*Actinomyces bovis* infection); listeriosis; botulism; thromboembolic meningoencephalitis; basilar empyema.

ii. The mouth should be examined after inserting a right Drinkwater gag and the alignment of the lower molar teeth on the left-hand side palpated. The diagnosis can be confirmed by radiography.

iii. The prognosis is good provided there is little displacement of the fracture. Intramuscular procaine penicillin is administered daily for 2–3 weeks to prevent infection of the fracture site.

iv. It is probable that the fracture was caused by trauma, possibly a tractor wheel, when the heifer had its head through the feed barrier.

59 A bright, alert 2-year-old Sim-
mental-cross beef heifer with
2 months' history of weight loss and
reduced appetite has developed
obvious brisket, submandibular, and
forelimb oedema (59a) over the past
2 weeks. The rectal temperature is
normal. The heifer has an increased
respiratory rate (30 breaths per minute) and is noted to eructate frequently. Auscultation of the chest
fails to reveal any abnormal lung
sounds but there is reduced reson-

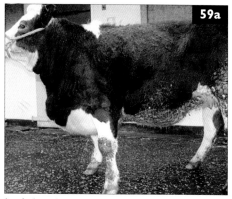

ance on percussion of the ventral third of the chest on both sides. The heart is
clearly audible with a rate of 72 beats per minute. Rumen motility is normal and
the heifer has passed normal faeces.
i. What conditions would you consider? (Most likely first.)
ii. How could you confirm your diagnosis?
iii. What action should you take?

60 During a routine fertility visit
you are presented with a calved
heifer for 'not seen bulling by
60 days' when you notice she has an
unusual pelvis (60). The farmer
reports that the heifer was unable to
rise for several days after she slipped
when entering the collecting yard
2 days after calving.
i. What conditions would you
consider?
ii. What action would you recommend?
iii. How could this problem have
been prevented?

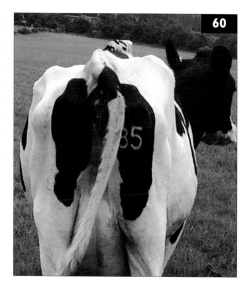

59 i. The most likely conditions to consider include: thymic lymphosarcoma causing compression of the cranial vena cava/oesophagus; right-sided heart failure caused by space-occupying mass in the thorax, e.g. large mediastinal abscess; dilated cardiomyopathy; septic pericarditis; chronic suppurative pneumonia/pleuritis/pleural effusion; endocarditis.

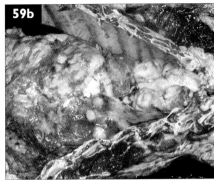

ii. Ultrasonography of the thorax reveals extensive pleural effusion accounting for the reduced resonance ventrally, however the mediastinum cannot be visualized. Thoracocentesis reveals a modified transudate; exfoliated tumour cells are rarely identified in cases of thymic lymphosarcoma. This examination does not rule out either a large mediastinal abscess or dilated cardiomyopathy. Serum protein concentrations are normal – there is unlikely to be significant long-standing bacterial infection. Dilated cardiomyopathy is not common in crossbred cattle.

iii. In the UK, concerns over infectious enzootic bovine leucosis virus require notification of regulatory authorities regarding suspicion of a tumour in cattle. The heifer was euthanased for welfare reasons and the diagnosis of thymic lymphosarcoma confirmed at necropsy (59b). Tests for enzootic bovine leucosis virus proved negative.

60 i. The most likely conditions to consider include: sacroiliac subluxation; previous fracture of the left wing of the ilium; trauma that has resulted in haematomata/abscess formation.

ii. There is no treatment for this condition. Sacroiliac subluxation should not cause an increased likelihood of dystocia because it does not significantly reduce the pelvic inlet.

iii. The farmer was advised to check for sudden right angle corners, narrow passageways, and other potential 'bottlenecks', and widen access for the cows as appropriate. Trauma to the wing of the ilium resulting in haematoma formation is not uncommon in dairy cattle. Narrow passageways and poorly designed cubicles are common causes of trauma causing haematoma formation. Bacterial infection of the haematoma(ta) may result in abscess formation in this area. Fractures of the wing of the ilium are not uncommon.

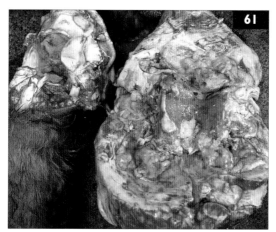

61 An 11-month-old beef stirk is presented for veterinary examination with marked lameness of several months' duration. The stirk is penned alone on deep straw bedding. The stirk is poorly grown and in body condition 2 (scale 1–5). The rectal temperature is 39.2°C (102.6°F). There is extensive soft tissue swelling surrounding the left hock region. The swelling is very firm, hot, and painful but there is no appreciable effusion of the hock joint. The popliteal lymph node is five times its normal size. There are no other swollen joints. The stirk should be euthanased immediately for welfare reasons. Both hock joints are examined at necropsy (**61**).

i. Was the decision to destroy this animal correct?

ii. What is the likely origin of this problem?

iii. What action should have been taken when the stirk was first noticed to be lame?

iv. What guidelines/instruction would you recommend to your clients?

62 A 20-month-old steer presents with sudden-onset severe bloat. The steer belongs to a group of 120 fattening cattle being fed a high production ration comprising *ad libitum* potatoes and maize gluten. The steer stands with its neck extended and head held lowered. The steer is salivating profusely and occasionally coughs up approximately 200 mL of saliva.

i. What conditions would you consider?

ii. What will you do?

61 i. Yes. There is almost complete destruction of joint cartilage into sub-chondral bone. There is extensive proliferation of the synovial membrane and fibrous tissue reaction surrounding the joint capsule. There is inspissated pus within the joint. It is estimated that the joint infection has been present for at least 3 months. The farmer has been negligent because this animal has suffered unnecessarily and has not received an appropriate level of care. Radiography often underestimates early joint pathology because much of the early reaction indicating the severity of lesion is comprised of soft tissue. However, at the stage illustrated here there would be extensive bone lysis and osteophyte reaction.
ii. The origin of infection is most likely a wound penetrating the joint. Bacteraemia localizing to one joint in growing cattle is unusual. There is no evidence of septic physitis extending into the joint.
iii. Veterinary examination is necessary for suspected joint infections. Treatment would include parenteral antibiotics and NSAIDs. Joint lavage will significantly improve the prognosis for recovery in many cases.
iv. Veterinary examination is essential when the cause of severe lameness is not immediately detected and corrected by the farmer, e.g. a sharp stone lodged in interdigital space causing necrobacillosis or white line separation causing an abscess. Such advice was obviously ignored in this case.

62 i. The most likely cause is choke (oesophageal obstruction). Rabies should be considered in countries where the disease is endemic.
ii. While a stomach tube can be passed to ascertain the position of the potato, this procedure simply wastes time. A probang is passed, but after approximately 60 cm along the cervical oesophagus the probang meets an obstruction. At this level the potato cannot be grasped by pushing your arm down the cow's oesophagus after inserting a Drinkwater mouth gag. Furthermore, the potato may be too large to push into the rumen without the risk of perforating the oesophagus.
   Instead a stainless steel fruit extractor is carefully inserted into the oesophagus until the loop contacts, and then slips over, the potato. The corkscrew is then extended into the potato by asking the farmer to turn the handle while you steady the steer's head. The potato is then removed. The steer immediately eructates a large amount of gas and forceful eructations can be heard over the next 5 minutes during which time the bloat is considerably reduced and the steer looks much happier.
   A rumen trochar is a last resort because it does not remove the obstruction. An obstruction such as a potato will not dissolve but it is likely to result in pressure necrosis of the oesophageal wall. In an emergency situation a trochar will relieve the bloat and allow slaughter of the steer.

63 A 3-year-old beef cow presents with 4 days' history of poor appetite and rapid weight loss. The cow had calved 10 days previously and had prolapsed her uterus immediately after delivery of a large dead calf that had been 'hip-locked'. The cow had received no antibiotics because the uterus was replaced easily and the placenta was already detached from the caruncles. The cow is now weak and depressed. The rectal temperature is 38.2°C (100.8°F). The ocular and oral mucous membranes appear slightly congested. The heart rate is 96 beats per minute. The respiratory rate is 30 breaths per minute with a slight abdominal component. The ruminal contractions are reduced and the cow has passed only scant faeces. Rectal examination reveals that the uterus is still extending well beyond the pelvic inlet. Vaginal examination reveals approximately 200 mL of foul-smelling brown fluid.

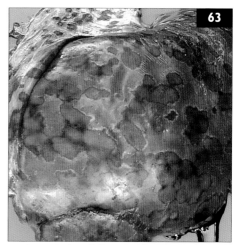

Despite treatment with intravenous oxytetracycline and flunixin for suspected metritis the cow died suddenly 2 days later. Postmortem examination reveals a septic metritis and the liver lesions shown in **63**.

i. What condition is affecting the liver?
ii. How could the provisional diagnosis be confirmed?
iii. Could this condition have been prevented?
iv. What is unusual about the aetiopathogenesis in this case?

64 i. Describe your analgesic regimen for a routine bovine caesarean operation.
ii. Are there any other drugs you could administer to assist surgery?
iii. Would you administer antibiotics?
iv. What suture material and suture pattern would you use for the uterus, abdominal wall, and skin?

63, 64: Answers

63 i. There are widespread severe *Fusobacterium necrophorum* lesions caused by local toxin production throughout the liver following bacteraemic spread from the uterus.

ii. *Fusobacterium necrophorum* can be cultured from the uterine contents and liver.

iii. It is rarely possibly to quantify the usefulness of prophylactic antibiotic therapy in large animal practice. Indeed, this practice is often questioned with respect to cost, food safety (milk and meat withdrawal periods), and selection for antibiotic resistance in certain bacterial species. However, in this particular case, prophylactic antibiotics after replacement of the uterine prolapse may well have prevented/cleared the uterine infection and/or prevented the bacteraemia seeding the liver with fatal consequences.

iv. *Fusobacterium necrophorum* is part of the normal rumen flora and hepatic lesions (encapsulated abscesses) often develop following grain overload/rumenitis and invasion via the portal circulation. No rumen lesions were detected in this cow.

64 i. Analgesia for a caesarean operation includes intravenous injection of a NSAID at least 5 minutes before surgery, with distal paravertebral anaesthesia using approximately 100 mL of 2% lidocaine. Xylazine (stages 3 and 4; animal would be recumbent) offers only 'a degree of analgesia' in data sheet information; no analgesia is afforded for standing surgery (stages 1 and 2). Sedation is not recommended for standing surgery because cattle may suddenly lie down during surgery with the associated risk of herniation of abdominal viscera through the flank incision.

ii. Clenbuterol can be administered to induce myometrial relaxation and aid manipulation of the uterus/calf. Oxytocin should be administered following surgery to stimulate uterine involution.

iii. There is no conclusive field trial regarding choice of antibiotic or route of administration to control bacterial infection. Intramuscular/intravenous antibiotic administration is recommended prior to surgery; intraperitoneal administration is frequently used after uterine closure. Intrauterine antibiotic pessaries are administered by some clinicians.

iv. The uterus is closed using an inversion suture (Cushing) of 7 metric chromic catgut. Some surgeons recommend two layers of uterine sutures for closure but this approach is often not possible due to the contracting uterus, nor is it necessary.

The abdominal wall is closed with two continuous suture layers of 7 metric chromic catgut: peritoneum and internal abdominal oblique muscle in the first layer, then the external abdominal oblique and transversus abdominis muscles in the second layer. The skin is closed with a Ford interlocking suture of monofilament nylon.

65 You are presented with a 5-month-old Limousin-cross beef calf, housed 2 weeks ago, which is dyspnoeic and stands with the neck extended, tongue protruded, and the head held in lowered position (65a). The rectal temperature is 41.1°C (106.0°F). There are no nasal or ocular discharges. The mucous membranes are congested. The respiratory rate is increased to

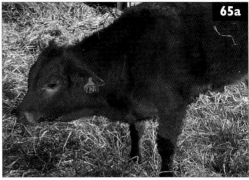

56 breaths per minute. There are reduced lungs sounds anteroventrally but crackles can be detected caudodorsally on auscultation. The remainder of the clinical examination is unremarkable. After handling, the calf's condition deteriorates further and it appears very distressed with flared nostrils and a marked abdominal component to respiration. An expiratory grunt can be heard for a short period after handling.

i. What conditions would you include in your differential diagnosis list?
ii. What treatment(s) would you administer?
iii. What control measures could be adopted for future years?

66 You are presented with a yearling Limousin-cross steer with a single large 50 cm diameter cutaneous lesion on the neck (66) which has been present for 6 months. The lesion is grey, firm, comprised of cornified epithelium, and deeply fissured, with a secondary bacterial infection producing a foul odour. The steer is afebrile, alert, and in good bodily con-

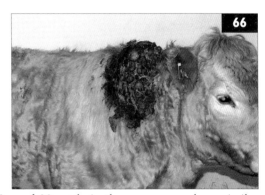

dition with a normal appetite. Two of 30 cattle in the same group have similar skin lesions on the brisket but they are less than 4–6 cm diameter.

i. What conditions would you consider?
ii. What is the likely cause?
iii. What control measures would you adopt?

65 i. The most likely conditions to consider include: peracute BRSV infection (with secondary bacterial infection); pasteurellosis; IBR infection; laryngeal diphtheresis (necrotic laryngitis); lungworm infestation.

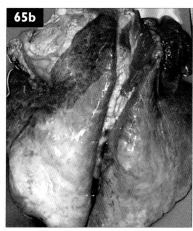

ii. Potential antibiotic treatments following secondary bacterial infection of BRSV-compromised lung defences include oxytetracycline, florfenicol, tilmicosin, taluthromycin, cefquinome, ceftiofur, and fluoroquinolone antibiotics.

A single injection of a soluble corticosteroid, such as dexamethasone, is indicated to reduce the immune-mediated/ allergic type reaction associated with inhalation of viral antigen into the caudodorsal lung (65b) in severe cases of BRSV-induced respiratory disease and may be life-saving. The benefits of NSAIDs, such as ketoprofen and flunixin meglumine, remain equivocal in such cases of severe respiratory disease.

iii. If proven to be the initiating cause (bronchoalveolar lavage, serology, FAT on lung section of any mortality) control is best achieved by vaccination against BRSV completed at least 2 weeks prior to housing.

The first clinical cases in a respiratory disease outbreak are typically the most severely affected, therefore veterinary attendance is essential at the start of any respiratory disease problem. Metaphylactic antibiotic administration is popular at the start of a respiratory disease outbreak to control secondary bacterial infection but there is little supporting evidence for efficacy in the veterinary literature.

66 i. The most likely conditions to consider include: papillomatosis (fibropapillomas, angleberries); other cutaneous neoplasms, including mast cell tumours or the cutaneous form of lymphosarcoma; skin tuberculosis; panniculitis; severe dermatophilosis.

ii. The likely cause is bovine papilloma virus.

iii. Control measures include isolation of affected cattle. These lesions usually spontaneously regress within 3–12 months. Crude autogenous vaccines can be used but the lesion(s) is often regressing by the stage this possibility is explored. The building should be thoroughly cleaned and disinfected before the next group of cattle are housed in it. The role of insect vectors in bovine papilloma virus transmission has been suggested but remains unproven. The lesion was slightly smaller when the steer was slaughtered 3 months later.

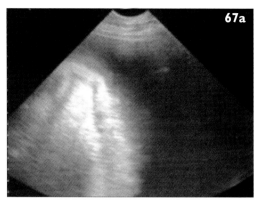

67 A 6-year-old Holstein cow presents with 2 weeks' history of poor appetite, weight loss, and poor milk yield. The cow has a painful facial expression, and walks slowly. The rectal temperature is elevated (39.2°C (102.6°F)). The heart rate is 80 beats per minute but the heart sounds are muffled on both sides of the chest. The respiratory rate is elevated to 40 breaths per minute with a slight abdominal component.
i. Describe the important features of the sonogram obtained at the sixth inter-costal space using a 5 MHz sector scanner (67a).
ii. How could you confirm your diagnosis?
iii. What action would you take?
iv. Could this situation have been prevented?

68 In late autumn a farmer reports the sudden death of a 6-year-old beef cow which calved 6 weeks ago. The cow is at pasture supplemented with 2 kg of barley per day but without added minerals/vitamins.
i. What conditions could cause sudden death in adult cattle? (Most likely first.)
ii. What action would you take?
iii. How could the cause of death be further investigated?
iv. What control measures could be adopted for the remainder of the herd?

67 i. Ultrasound examination reveals 5–6 cm fluid (anechoic area) distension of the pericardial sac. There is 2 cm fibrin deposition on the epicardium (broad irregular hyperechoic band) and oedema of the myocardium (narrow anechoic band underlying the fibrin deposits). These findings are consistent with a diagnosis of septic pericarditis (**67b**).

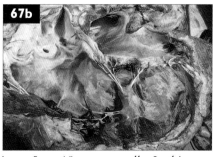

ii. Pericardiocentesis can be carried out using a 5 cm 18-gauge needle. In this case pericardiocentesis yielded a turbid, yellow–brown, foul-smelling fluid – pus.
iii. There is no effective treatment of septic pericarditis and the cow should be euthanased immediately for welfare reasons. While pericardial strips are described in the literature, they are never performed in general practice. Removal of the fibrin deposits on the epicardium would not be possible in this case. At necropsy a 7 cm piece of wire extended through the left ventricular wall into the heart chamber (**67b**).
iv. Septic pericarditis occurs in some cases of traumatic reticulitis following penetration of the pericardial sac by a sharp metal object. Routine administration of magnets to lodge within the reticulum is practised in herds with a history of 'hardware disease' to attract and bind ingested metal objects.

68 i. The most likely causes of sudden death include: hypomagnesaemia; lightning strike; anthrax; clostridial diseases such as blackleg.
ii. The farmer must inform the regulatory authority (Divisional Veterinary Manager in the UK). A blood smear is then collected by the veterinarian and tested for anthrax (*Bacillus anthracis*) using McFadyean's methylene blue stain.
iii. In anthrax-negative cases, further investigations could include collection of aqueous humour (or cisternal CSF) for magnesium concentration, with around 0.1 mmol/L (0.2 mEq/L) consistent with profound hypomagnesaemia before death. Blood samples may be taken from four to six cows in the group, where magnesium concentrations below 0.5 mmol/L (1 mEq/L) are a warning of potential clinical hypomagnesaemia.
iv. Control measures could include replacing the 2 kg of barley with high-magnesium concentrates. The cows should also be offered *ad libitum* roughage; straw will suffice. Free-access minerals are an unreliable source of daily magnesium intake.

69 Analgesia after lumbosacral extradural injection of 3 mg/kg of 2% lidocaine has numerous applications in cattle practice.
i. List the uses of lumbosacral extradural injection.
ii. How is this procedure undertaken?
iii. What is the duration of effective analgesia following this procedure?

70 A very valuable 5-year-old Limousin bull has been unable to serve six cows presented to him over the previous 4 weeks. The bull has mounted the cows with the penis extruded for about 20 cm but failed to enter the vagina and thrust normally. He has failed to produce normal semen when collected by artificial vagina on two occasions 1 month apart. The bull had previously sired calves by natural service for three breeding seasons, and no less than 10 months prior to veterinary examination.

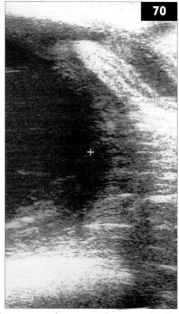

On examination, the bull is sound, bright, and alert, and presents in excellent body condition with a normal appetite. The rectal temperature is 38.5°C (101.3°F). The bull has passed normal quantities of faeces but drips urine almost continually from the prepuce. There are no signs of colic, tenesmus, or pumping of the tail. Anal and tail tone, and perineal skin sensation are normal. There are no abnormalities of the external genitalia. Manual rectal examination reveals a markedly distended urinary bladder extending cranially for more than 40 cm (arm's length) from the pelvic brim. Ultrasound examination using a 5 MHz linear probe shows the bladder distended beyond the 10 cm scanner range (70) and containing increased amounts of cast material (sabulous concretions). There is no pulsation in the pelvic urethra. Immediate microsopic examination of three ejaculates reveals no gross motility. Nigrosin and eosin-stained semen preparations demonstrate no live sperm, 51% with detached heads, 8% with bent mid-pieces, and 11% with simple bent tails.
i. List the differential diagnoses you would consider for the bladder distension?
ii. What is the prognosis for this bull's future fertility?
iii. What is the likely aetiology?

69, 70: Answers

69 i. Lumbosacral extradural injection can provide surgical analgesia for: examination/repair pelvic limb fractures; examination/flushing pelvic limb joints; tibial neurectomy (treatment for spastic paresis); vasectomy; penile and urethral surgery (sacrococcygeal site is adequate for subischial urethrostomy).

ii. The animal is carefully restrained in sternal recumbency. The lumbosacral site is identified as the midline depression midway between the last palpable lumbar dorsal spine (L6) and the first palpable sacral dorsal spine (S2). The site is clipped, surgically prepared, and a small amount of local anaesthetic solution injected subcutaneously. The needle is advanced at a right angle to the vertebral column through skin, subcutaneous tissue, supraspinous and interarcuate ligaments, and ligamentum flavum into the dorsal extradural space (40–60 kg, 25 mm 20-gauge; 65–100 kg, 38 mm 19-gauge; 100–200 kg, 50 mm 19-gauge needle). The needle is advanced slowly over 5–10 s to appreciate the 'pop through' the interarcuate ligament. At this point the negative pressure will draw the drop of saline down from the needle hub ('hanging drop' test). If the needle point enters the subarachnoid space, CSF will collect in the needle hub within 2–3 s, thereafter the dose rate of lidocaine must be reduced to one third of the original calculation.

iii. The duration of analgesia/paralysis of the pelvic limbs is up to 4 hr.

70 i. The most likely conditions to consider include: pelvic nerve damage; partial urolithiasis. The sacral part of the parasympathetic outflow constitutes the pelvic nerves with postganglionic neurons found within the walls of the descending colon, rectum, accessory sex glands, genital erectile tissue, and bladder. Damage to the spinal cord above the sacral nerves (upper motor neuron tracts) or the sacral cord and nerves supplying the detrusor muscle (lower motor neuron tracts) may result in urinary incontinence. Normal pelvic limb function and absence of cauda equina syndrome in this bull would exclude upper motor neuron tracts and sacral segment involvement, respectively.

ii. The prognosis for return of acceptable fertility in this bull is guarded because of the absence of live sperm in the samples collected and very high percentage of defects, although detached normal heads and simple bent tails are classified as minor defects.

iii. While sacral fractures are not uncommon in adult bulls, there was no evidence of cauda equina syndrome in this case. For the same reason, lymphosarcoma was excluded from the list of possible aetiologies. Other causes of pelvic nerve dysfunction, such as protozoal myelitis, were considered but could not be proven. The aetiology of the suspected pelvic nerve dysfunction in this bull was not determined.

71 Describe how you would remove a sharp metal object from the reticulum of a dairy cow (traumatic reticulitis/hardware surgery). Pay particular attention to:
i. Anaesthesia and analgesia.
ii. Exteriorization of the rumen and entering the reticulum.
iii. Finding the object in the reticular wall.
iv. Closing the rumenotomy.

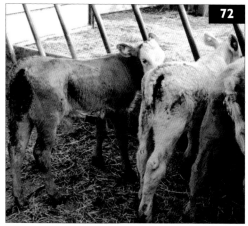

72 During hot summer weather you are presented with a group of 3-month-old single suckled beef calves that have been grazing a 25 hectare field. The only water supply is a small stream which has almost dried up; there is a lot of poaching and faecal contamination of the ground surrounding the edges of the stream. Several calves have profuse diarrhoea, containing mucus and small flecks of fresh blood, with considerable staining of the perineum and tail (72). Tenesmus with partial eversion of the rectum is observed in two calves. The clinical signs are less marked in the remaining calves where chronic wasting and poor appetite are the presenting signs. The rectal temperatures are normal.
i. What conditions would you consider? (Most likely first.)
ii. How would you confirm your diagnosis?
iii. What treatment(s) would you recommend?
iv. What control measures could be adopted?

71 i. Analgesia is afforded by flunixin or other NSAID injected intravenously at least 5 minutes prior to surgery. High left flank laporotomy is performed under distal paravertebral analgesia.

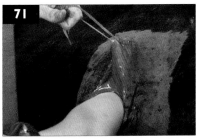

ii. Two 5 mm nylon tape loops are placed 15 cm apart in the muscular layer of the rumen following its exteriorization. The rumen wall is incised between the tape loops. The rumen is pulled on to the surgeon's right arm while the assistant holds the tape loops (71). The surgeon's arm passes through 8–10 cm crust of fibrous rumen content before entering rumen liquor. The hand is angled towards the xiphisternum taking the rumen back in through the abdominal incision site (if it is a large cow) provided that the rumen incision fits tightly around the arm and there is no leakage which could contaminate the peritoneum. The hand is passed along the rumen floor then upward and forward into the reticulum.

iii. The 'honeycomb' lining of the reticulum is searched carefully for the foreign body. Checks are made for serosal adhesions by picking up a fold of reticulum wall. The reticular wall will be oedematous (thickened) and adherent to adjacent structures where the foreign body has penetrated.

iv. The rumen incision is closed with a Connell suture of 3 metric chromic catgut. The abdominal wall muscles are closed using two layers of continuous catgut sutures. A Ford interlocking pattern using nylon is used to close the skin. Antibiotics, such as penicillin, are given daily for 3–5 consecutive days following surgery.

72 i. The most likely conditions to consider include: coccidiosis (*Eimeria alabamensis*); salmonellosis; PGE (ostertigosis type I); lead poisoning; ragwort poisoning. If only one calf was affected then one could also consider intus-susception and necrotic enteritis.

ii. A diagnosis of coccidiosis can be made based upon clinical findings and supported by a high oocyst count in the faecal samples collected from six calves. Faecal oocyst counts can be highly variable and *Eimeria* speciation should be undertaken. Response to treatment is also a helpful indirect diagnostic aid.

iii. The treatment is diclazuril administered to all calves. Multivitamin injections may help convalescence in debilitated calves.

iv. Control measures include moving the cows and calves from the infected pastures to another field. Advice should be given about installing a mains water supply. In pastured cattle during hot dry summer weather, reliance on small streams to provide water can lead to rapid faecal contamination of the water/surrounding pasture causing clinical coccidiosis in susceptible calves.

73 You are presented with a 2-year-old Holstein heifer that has developed obvious brisket, submandibular, and forelimb oedema over the past 3 weeks (73a). The rectal temperature is normal. The heifer has an increased respiratory rate (54 breaths per minute) with frequent nonproductive coughing. Auscultation of the chest reveals reduced audibility of lung sounds and reduced resonance on percussion of the ventral third on both sides of the chest. The heart sounds can only be heard from the left hind side of the chest. The heart rate is 90 beats per

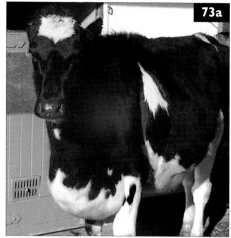

minute and regular. The jugular veins are markedly distended. There is no lameness and there are no palpable joint distensions.
i. What conditions would you consider? (Most likely first.)
ii. What further investigations would you undertake?
iii. What action/treatment would you recommend?

74 A dairy farmer complains that a high proportion of his cows have large scaly skin lesions either side of the root of the tail (perianal fossae) (74). The lesions have become much more prevalent during the last month. The lesions are nonpruritic and there is no localized erythema.
i. What conditions would you consider?
ii. Which further tests could be undertaken?
iii. What actions/treatments would you recommend?

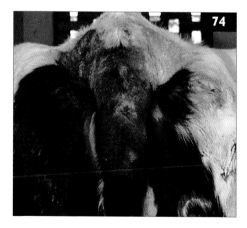

73, 74: Answers

73 i. The most likely conditions to consider include: Holstein dilated cardiomyopathy; right-sided heart failure caused by space-occupying mass in the thorax, e.g. a large mediastinal abscess or thymic lymphosarcoma; myocarditis; pericarditis; chronic suppurative pneumonia/pleuritis/pleural effusion; hypoproteinaemia (caused by chronic liver disease) resulting in peripheral oedema; endocarditis.

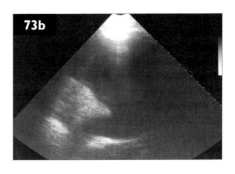

ii. Further investigations could include haematological examination and ultrasonographic examination of the chest. Routine haematological examination reveals normal values for total red blood cell count (7.6×10^{12}/L (7.6×10^6/µL), range 5–9 $\times 10^{12}$/L (5–9 $\times 10^6$/µL)) and haemoglobin (112 g/L (11.2 g/dL), range 80–140 g/L (8–14 g/dL)). There is a normal white cell count (5.1×10^9/L (5.1×10^3/µL), range 4–10 $\times 10^9$/L (4–10 $\times 10^3$/µL)) comprised of 58% neutrophils and 36% lymphocytes. There is a slight hypoalbuminaemia and moderate hypoglobulinaemia (24 g/L (2.4 g/dL) and 29.3 g/L (2.93 g/dL), respectively). The AST concentration is slightly increased (147 IU/L; normal 53–105 IU/L). There is no haematological evidence of chronic inflammation and the albumin concentration is not compatible with oedema from low plasma oncotic pressure.

Ultrasonography reveals an extensive pleural effusion occupying the ventral half of the chest with dorsal displacement of the lung (73b). Thoracocentesis yields pale straw-coloured fluid with the characteristics of a transudate; there are no exfoliated tumour cells.

iii. The heifer should be euthanased for welfare reasons. Holstein dilated cardiomyopathy affects 2–4-year-old animals and an inherited aetiology has been suggested. Diagnosis is based upon exclusion of other possible aetiologies of right-sided heart failure, although an increased heart rate and dysrhythmia are common findings.

74 i. The most likely conditions to consider include: chorioptic mange; lice (pediculosis); sarcoptic mange; ringworm (*Trichophyton* spp. infection); dermatophilosis.

ii. The lesions are typical of chorioptic mange which rarely causes lesions in other areas of the body. Microscopic examination of skin scrapings yields an occasional *Chorioptes bovis* mite. Pediculosis is a much more generalized infestation and examination of the skin with the naked eye would reveal lice.

iii. No treatment is necessary in this situation because the lesions are mild and typically regress following turnout to pasture.

75 A 4-month-old beef suckler calf presents with marked lameness (9/10) of 3 weeks' duration, and soft tissue swelling over the left distal metatarsal/fetlock joint region (75a). The calf is well grown and in good body condition. The rectal temperature is 39.2°C (102.6°F). The swelling is hot and painful and extends proximally beyond the proximal extent of the fetlock joint. There is no obvious effusion of the fetlock joint. The popliteal lymph node cannot be palpated. There are no other swollen joints. No other significant clinical abnormalities are detected.

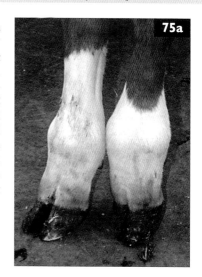

i. What conditions would you consider?
ii. How would you confirm your diagnosis?
iii. What action would you take?

76 A 30 kg 5-day-old Charolais-cross twin bull calf from a beef herd is dull and unwilling to suck its dam. The calf is reluctant to rise but can stand when assisted to its feet (76). The calf has sunken eyes and the skin tent is extended to 4 s. The rectal temperature is 39.6°C (103.3°F). The mucous membranes are congested and there is episcleral congestion. The respiratory rate is increased at 30 breaths per minute.

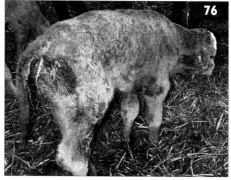

The heart rate is 120 beats per minute. The abdomen is shrunken with little content in the abomasum/intestines and there is mild diarrhoea. There is slight thickening of the umbilical stump. The joints and carcass lymph nodes are not enlarged. The co-twin appears normal. The cow has chronic mastitis in two quarters that are not functional.

i. What conditions would you consider?
ii. What tests would you undertake to support your provisional diagnosis?
iii. What treatment(s) would you administer?
iv. What control measures would you recommend?

75, 76: Answers

75 i. The most likely conditions to consider include: infected fracture of the distal growth plate of the third metatarsal bone; fracture of the third metatarsal bone; septic metatarsophalangeal (fetlock) following puncture wound; cellulitis/tendon sheath infection.

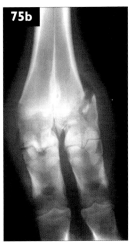

ii. Arthrocentesis is not attempted because there is no obvious joint effusion. Furthermore, experience has shown that because of the extensive synovial membrane proliferation and fibrinous nature of the bovine inflammatory response, joint fluid can rarely be aspirated from chronically infected bovine joints. Lateromedial and dorsoplantar radiographs of the left fetlock region reveal marked soft tissue swelling with an infected Salter-Harris type III fracture of the distal third metatarsal bone (75b). There is also widening of the joint space and irregularity of the articular surfaces of the left fetlock joint indicating extension of infection distally. Ruminants are frequently bacteraemic and infection of fracture sites is not uncommon.

iii. The calf should be euthanased because of the grave prognosis.

76 i. The most likely conditions to consider include: septicaemia associated with failure of passive antibody transfer; early bacterial meningoencephalitis; starvation and diarrhoea caused by nonenterotoxigenic *Escherichia coli* strains; enterotoxigenic *Escherichia coli*.

ii. Early bacterial meningoencephalitis could be excluded by visual examination of lumbar CSF collected under local anaesthesia using a 20-gauge 25 mm hypodermic needle; normal CSF is clear and colourless. Determination of total plasma protein concentration in the practice laboratory using a refractometer reveals a concentration of 46 g/L (4.6 g/dL) consistent with failure of passive transfer (normal >65 g/L, >6.5 g/dL).

iii. Treatment for septicaemia could include intravenous administration of trimethoprim/sulphonamide and ketoprofen (a NSAID). The calf was also treated with an oral rehydration solution offered by teat (1 L every 2 hr). An orogastric tube can be used but is a less useful guide to the calf's condition/demeanour. This calf made a full recovery.

iv. Failure of passive antibody transfer and a heavily contaminated environment predispose neonates to septicaemia/bacteraemia. All newborn calves must receive colostrum equivalent to 7% of their bodyweight within the first 6 hr of life. Colostrum must also be stored in the deep freeze for those situations when the cow calves without sufficient good-quality colostrum.

77 A 3-week-old beef suckler calf was found one morning by the farmer with sudden-onset foreleg lameness and swelling of the elbow joint. Your client suspected an injury from the bull running with the group of cows but nonetheless decided to inject the calf with long-acting oxytetracycline at 20 mg/kg. The calf's condition deteriorated and you are presented with the calf 3 weeks later. The calf is bright and alert but it is

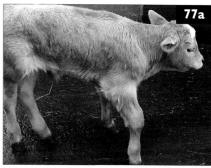

9/10 lame on the right foreleg (77a) and is also lame on the left hindleg. The rectal temperature is 39.7°C (103.5°F). The mucous membranes appear normal. The right elbow joint is hot, swollen, and painful on gentle palpation. The right prescapular lymph node is markedly enlarged. The left fore fetlock is hot, swollen, and painful on gentle palpation. The left prescapular lymph node is also markedly enlarged. The left stifle joint is hot, swollen, and painful on gentle palpation. The left hind fetlock joint is hot, swollen, and painful on gentle palpation with enlargement of the popliteal lymph node.
i. What conditions would you consider?
ii. What action would you take?

78 A 2.5-year-old Holstein heifer presents with anorexia, marked drop in milk yield, and profuse salivation. Other cattle in the group are less severely affected and the farmer suspects the caustic action of ammonia-treated straw added to the total mixed ration for the first time 3 days ago. The heifer's rectal temperature is 40.5°C (104.9°F). There is ulceration of dental pad and hard palate (78). The submucosa is markedly

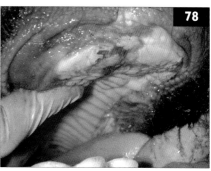

hyperaemic with sloughing of the overlying epithelium over a large area. There is increased salivation. There are no ocular or nasal discharges.
i. What conditions would you consider? (Most likely first.)
ii. What other clinical signs would you check for?
iii. What action would you take?
iv. What samples would you collect to confirm your provisional diagnosis?
v. What control measures would you recommend?

77 i. The only likely condition to consider is septic polyarthritis. Arthrocentesis yielded less than 1 mL of turbid joint fluid from the elbow joint. There was insufficent sample for total white cell and differential counts. Radiography of the left fore fetlock (77b) confirms the diagnosis of sepsis with extensive bony proliferation and possible osteomyelitis.

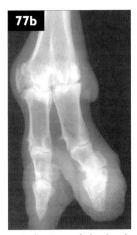

ii. All cases of lameness in calves less than 8 weeks of age should be considered septic unless proven otherwise. The choice of antibiotic can prove difficult and many clinicians elect to administer amoxicillin/clavulanic acid combination for 10 consecutive days. Florfenicol is also commonly used for polyarthritis in young calves. Joint lavage can be successful if only one joint is affected. A recent study reported an 80% response to joint lavage, although the majority of cases required two or more flushes. Infection of the hock joint carried the best prognosis, those cases with infection of the stifle joint the worst. The calf shown here was euthanased for welfare reasons.

78 i. The most likely conditions to consider include: foot and mouth disease; MD; malignant catarrhal fever; bluetongue.
ii. Other clinical signs of foot and mouth disease to check for include vesicles progressing to ulceration of the interdigital space and coronary band. Other cattle in the group should be examined. Farm records should be checked for animal and vehicle movements.
iii. Immediate action would include informing the Police and Divisional Veterinary Manager of Animal Health (formerly State Veterinary Service) in the UK. The appropriate regulatory authorities must be informed as necessary in other countries. Do not leave the premises and stop all movement of people, vehicles, and animals on to and off the premises.
iv. Contents of vesicles and 2 cm^2 overlying mucosal flap and a blood sample must be collected.
v. Control measures for foot and mouth disease are determined nationally. Slaughter of all cloven-hooved animals on the farm with full compensation operated in the UK during the 2001 foot and mouth disease epidemic. The 3 km contiguous cull proved very contentious especially in Scotland during this outbreak. The 2007 outbreak of foot and mouth disease in the UK was traced to poor biosecurity measures at a research laboratory. Slaughter of all cloven-hooved animals on the affected farms with full compensation again operated but there was no contiguous cull. Ring vaccination was considered but not used, presumably due to the known origin of the infection.

79 A 9-month-old (340 kg) Holstein bull, which has been dull and inappetant for the past 2 days, presents with a large swelling of the ventral abdomen which extends from the scrotum to the prepuce (79). The bull often adopts a wide stance with the hindlimbs placed further back than normal. There is frequent bruxism (teeth grinding). The rectal temperature is normal (38.5°C (101.3°F)).

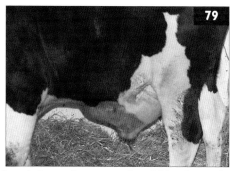

The bull stands with the tail head raised and shows frequent tail swishing but only a few drops of urine rather than a continous flow are voided. The drops of urine are slightly blood-tinged. There are numerous calculi on the preputial hairs. The swelling of the ventral abdominal wall pits under pressure.
i. What conditions would you consider?
ii. What further clinical examination should be undertaken?
iii. How would you correct this problem?
iv. What control measures could be adopted?

80 A 5-year-old Holstein cow, which calved 1 month ago and was previously yielding 42 L/day, presents with a poor appetite and milk yield which has fallen steadily over the past 2 days to 22 L/day. The cow has been licking at objects such as walls and her own flanks for long periods of time. The rectal temperature is normal. The cow has a gaunt appearance with sunken sublumbar fossae consistent with a reduced appetite (80). The cow is constipated while other cows in the high-yielding group have soft faeces.

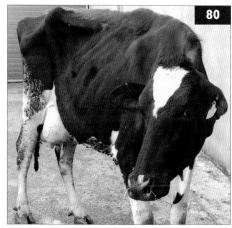

i. What conditions would you consider? (Most likely first.)
ii. How could you confirm your diagnosis?
iii. What treatment would you administer?
iv. How could this condition be prevented?

79, 80: Answers

79 i. The most likely conditions to consider include: partial obstructive urolithiasis/ruptured urethra with subcutaneous urine accumulation; ruptured penis and haematoma formation; cellulitis from puncture wound of the ventral abdomen wall; infectious balanoposthitis.

ii. Rectal examination reveals a massively distended bladder and pulsations within the urethra consistent with urolithiasis. The BUN concentration is elevated at 22.8 mmol/L (63.8 mg/dL) (normal range 2–6 mmol/L, 5.6–16.8 mg/dL).

iii. Cattle, unlike sheep, are not prone to developing hydronephrosis following partial/complete urethral obstruction. Surgery is employed as a salvage procedure to enable the bull to overcome the uraemia and put on condition over the next few months before being slaughtered. Surgical correction of urolithiasis involves a subischial urethrostomy under caudal block. The penis is bluntly dissected distally then transected to reflect 10 cm above the skin level. Infection of the sectioned urethra almost invariably occurs after surgery, causing first cystitis then pyelonephritis with clinical signs apparent around 6–8 weeks following surgery.

iv. There are no specific control measures. In young calves urolithiasis has been associated with bladder infection arising from an infected urachus. Urolithiasis occurs sporadically in single intensively fed cattle, more often in bulls than in castrated males.

80 i. The most likely conditions to consider include: nervous acetonaemia/ketosis; left-displaced abomasum and secondary acetonaemia; traumatic reticulitis; subacute ruminal acidosis.

ii. Diagnosis of ketosis is based on clinical examination and confirmed by a positive Rothera's reagent test or laboratory demonstration of a 3-OH butyrate concentration in excess of 4.0 mmol/L (40 mg/dL). Plasma glucose and NEFA concentrations are too variable to confirm a diagnosis of ketosis. No biochemical test differentiates between primary and secondary ketosis. It must be ascertained that the cow does not have a left-displaced abomasum.

iii. Treatment includes dexamethasone and 400mL 50% dextrose administered intravenously. Propylene glycol is given orally twice daily until normal appetite returns. The cow was eating well the following day.

iv. Control measures include feeding molasses-treated chopped straw as part of the ration during the dry period to maintain rumen size and microbial function. Dry matter intakes should be as high as possible during the dry period, and on the day of calving in particular. There must be 24 hr of easy access to the diet – one should not rely on feeding refusals from the milking herd ration to the dry cows. Any dietary changes must be introduced gradually. Most high-yielding cows are fed a total mixed ration which has the benefit of creating a more stable rumen environment than that achieved with separate concentrate feeding. Cows should enter the dry period in BCS 3 (scale 1–5) and maintain that value until calving.

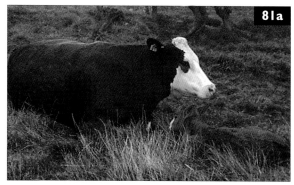

81 During late summer you are presented with a recumbent 7-year-old Limousin-cross-Friesian beef cow which calved unaided 12 hr earlier. The cow is in sternal recumbency (**81a**), depressed, afebrile (38.5°C (101.3°F)), with normal mucous membranes, a heart rate of 76 beats per minute, and a normal respiratory rate (20 breaths per minute). There is mild ruminal bloat. No abnormalities can be detected by palpation of the udder or stripping all four quarters. The cow makes several feeble attempts to rise but is unable to raise her body off the ground.
i. Which diseases would you consider? (Most likely first.)
ii. What treatment(s) would you administer?
iii. How could this condition be controlled/prevented?

82 This sample has been collected by abdominocentesis immediately caudal to the xiphisternum from a cow with suspected peritonitis associated with traumatic reticulitis.

The results of a peritoneal fluid sample are shown.

Total protein	76.5 g/L (7.65 g/dL)	
White cells	55.7 × 10⁹/L	
	(55.7 × 10³/µL)	
Cytology	Neutrophils	99%
	Lymphocytes	1%

i. What technique would assist peritoneal fluid collection?
ii. Comment upon the sample analysis.
iii. What other haematological/biochemical analyses could be undertaken?
iv. What other tests could be undertaken for traumatic reticulitis?

81, 82: Answers

81 i. The most likely conditions to consider include: hypocalcaemia; hypomagnesaemia; environmental mastitis; other infectious conditions causing toxaemia/endotoxaemia; trauma at parturition with either ruptured uterus/peritonitis or severe haemorrhage.

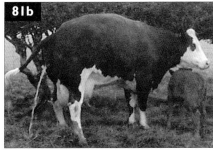

ii. Treatment includes intravenous administration of 400 mL of 40% calcium borogluconate given slowly over 10 minutes with the heart rate monitored throughout infusion. Typically, the animal will eructate after several minutes, pass faeces towards the end of the infusion, attempt to stand 5–10 minutes later, and urinate once standing (81b). As an insurance policy 400 mL of 40% calcium borogluconate is often injected subcutaneously but calcium salts are poorly absorbed from this site, are irritant to local tissue, and painful. Recurrence of hypocalcaemia is very uncommon in beef cows.

iii. Hypocalcaemia occurs sporadically in older beef cows (fourth lactation and beyond). Diet manipulation (dietary cation/anion balance) is not a realistic means of controlling hypocalcaemia in beef cattle. Feeding high-magnesium cobs may correct marginal hypomagnesaemia and thereby help reduce hypocalcaemia but such a feeding regimen may not be practicable.

82 i. Ultrasonographic examination immediately caudal to the xiphisternum typically reveals large quantities of inflammatory exudate in early cases of peritonitis, facilitating sample collection.

ii. There is an increased protein concentration (>30 g/L, >3.0 g/dL), and elevated white cell count (>3.0 × 10^9/L, >3.0 × 10^3/µL) comprised almost entirely of neutrophils consistent with an inflammatory exudate.

iii. Routine haematological examination in this cow reveals mild anaemia: total red blood cell count 4.6 × 10^{12}/L (4.6 × 10^6/µL) (normal range 5–9 × 10^{12}/L, 5–9 × 10^6/µL); haemoglobin 85 g/L (8.5 g/dL) (normal range 80–140 g/L, 8–14 g/dL), and a packed cell volume of 0.24 L/L (normal range 0.24–0.34 L/L). There is a marked leucocytosis (17.2 × 10^9/L (17.2 × 10^3/µL), normal range 4–10 × 10^9/L, 4–10 × 10^3/µL), comprised of 87% neutrophils, with 3% immature neutrophils and 10% lymphocytes. There is a markedly increased haptoglobin concentration (2.02 g/L (0.202 g/dL), normal <0.1 g/L, <0.01g/dL) indicating acute bacterial infection. There is a profound hypoalbuminaemia and high globulin concentration (16 g/L (1.6 g/dL) and 50.5 g/L (5.05 g/dL), respectively) consistent with a chronic severe bacterial infection.

iv. Radiography is costly and is not an option in most large animal practices. Metal detectors are a waste of time in the diagnosis of traumatic reticulitis because there are often many harmless pieces of metal in the reticulum.

83 A collapsed 10-day-old, 45 kg beef calf (83a) presents with profuse diarrhoea of 3 days' duration. The calf is unresponsive and very weak despite treatment with an oral rehydration solution twice daily by the farmer. The eyes are not sunken and the skin tent duration is normal. There is no episcleral injection. The rectal temperature is 38.0°C (100.4°F). The heart

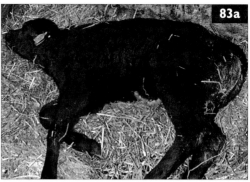

rate is 82 beats per minute. The respiratory rate is 30 breaths per minute. The umbilicus is not swollen. No joints swellings can be detected.

i. What is your diagnosis?

ii. What treatments would you administer?

iii. What control measures should be implemented?

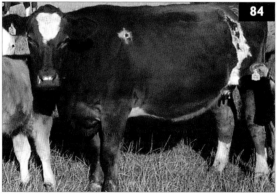

84 A 5-year-old cow presents with skin lesions confined to the nonpigmented areas (84). The affected skin is dry and raised at the periphery from normal healthy pigmented skin. The skin of the teats appears dry and 'papery'. The farmer also reports that this cow often has a red nose during the summer.

i. What conditions would you consider? (Most likely first.)

ii. What are the possible causes?

iii. What advice would you offer?

83 i. The clinical signs of profound depression and weakness following a period of severe diarrhoea are consistent with acidosis caused rotavirus/corona-virus infection. There is no evidence of septicaemia such as injected scleral vessels, fever, or other organ system involvement such as polyarthritis, pneumonia, panophthalmitis or meningitis.

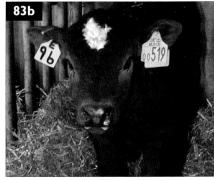

ii. Treatment must correct the acidosis. The calf is estimated to be no more than 5% dehydrated. Fluid replacement requirements are 45 kg × 0.05 = 2 L plus daily requirement of 75–150 mL/kg (equal to 3–6 L/day). The base deficit for recumbent/stuporous calves is estimated to be 20 mmol/L. The total base deficit (or negative base excess) is calculated as:

$$\text{base deficit} \times \text{bicarbonate space} \times \text{dehydrated calf weight}$$
$$= 20 \times (0.5) \times 40 = 400 \text{ mmol bicarbonate (400 mEq)}$$
$$16\text{g sodium bicarbonate} = 200 \text{ mmol of bicarbonate}$$

16 g sodium bicarbonate (200 mmol bicabonate) are dissolved in 1 L of isotonic saline and infused over the first 20 minutes and the remaining 200 mmol bicarbonate are dissolved in 3 L and given over the next 3 hr.

Oral fluids should be offered at a rate of 1 L eight times daily. A bottle and teat is preferred to an orogastric tube to gauge the calf's mental state and appetite (83b). This calf was not treated with antibiotics.

iii. All cows should be vaccinated with rotavirus/coronavirus vaccine when such aetiology is confirmed. Passive antibody transfer should be ensured. The remaining pregnant cows should be moved to a clean environment.

84 i. The most likely conditions are: photosensitization; dermatophilosis.

ii. Primary photosensitization occurs when preformed photodynamic agents are absorbed from the gastrointestinal tract. Hepatogenous photosensitization results from the liver disease and the inability to excrete phylloerythrin, a metabolite of chlorophyll. Liver disease and secondary photosensitization can be caused by the ingestion of mouldy feed containing aflatoxins.

iii. The cow should be housed to protect the animal from direct sunlight. Systemic corticosteroids may be indicated in the acute erythematous stage of photo-sensitization to prevent extensive inflammation and necrosis but this stage had long passed and the cow was 6 months pregnant (risk of abortion). Topical emollients and antimicrobials may help soften and protect the skin.

85 You are presented with a 6-year-old Friesian cow which is dull and depressed (**85a**). The cow is yielding only 18 L/day when normally 40–45 L/day would be expected 3 weeks after calving. Clinical examination reveals a normal rectal temperature. The cow is slightly constipated. A sweet ketotic smell is obvious on the cow's breath. Normal rumen movements can be heard caudally in

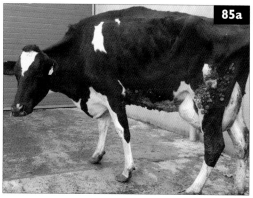

the sublumbar fossa. On percussion, high-pitched metallic sounds ('ping, ping, ping') can be heard high up on the left-hand side under the ribs. Rectal examination fails to reveal any abnormality. There is no evidence of mastitis.

i. What is your diagnosis?

ii. What other conditions could cause tympany in this area?

iii. What action would you take?

iv. What treatment(s) would you administer?

86 You are presented with a 6-year-old pedigree Aberdeen Angus beef cow with a cervico-vaginal prolapse (**86**). The cow calved unaided 2 days previously and passed the placenta within 2 hr.

i. How would you correct this problem?

ii. What is your advice regarding the management of this cow?

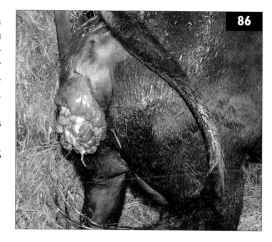

85 i. The LDA occupies the cranio-dorsal area of the left side of the abdominal cavity where auscultation and succusion reveals high-pitched 'tinkling' sounds. There is also evidence of secondary ketosis.

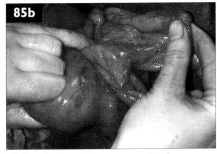

ii. Other conditions that cause high-pitched metallic sounds on the left side of the abdomen include rumen void, which refers to the gap caused by the shrunken rumen falling away from the left abdominal wall, a gas cap in the rumen associated with ruminal atony, acidosis/grain overload, and pneumoperitoneum.

iii. There are numerous treatment options. Rolling the cow to correct the LDA has been practised but requires three people, is almost as time consuming as surgery, and less than 40% successful. Surgery is performed in the standing cow under distal paravertebral analgesia. A right laporotomy incision is made and the abomasum deflated using a 14-gauge needle connected to a flutter valve. Upon release of gas, the abomasum slowly sinks towards the ventral midline pulled by its liquid contents. The greater omentum is grasped by the surgeon and pulled around to the ventral margin of the right laporotomy incision. An omentopexy (85b) or pyloropexy is performed: a continuous suture taking four 2 cm bites of omentum or pylorus is continued to close the peritoneum and internal oblique muscle layer. The laparotomy wound is then closed routinely.

iv. Treatment for the secondary acetonaemia comprises an intramuscular injection of dexamethasone and 400 mL of 50% dextrose administered intravenously.

86 i. The vaginal prolapse is replaced after sacrococcygeal extradural injection of 5 mL of 2% lidocaine. Note that the needle should be advanced at 45° to the vertebral column. The prolapsed tissues are thoroughly cleaned in warm dilute antiseptic solution. Steady pressure should be applied to the prolapsed tissues. A Buhner suture of 5 mm umbilical tape is placed in the subcutaneous tissue surrounding the vulva.

ii. The farmer should be advised of the high probability of recurrence after subsequent calving. In natural mating systems cows can become pregnant despite the Buhner retention suture *in situ*. Should this happen the suture must be slackened before the expected calving date. The suture can be retied after calving and passage of the fetal membranes. Vaginal prolapse is more commonly encountered 1–3 months after calving, most commonly during oestrus and following mounting another cow.

87 A 4-month-old Charolais beef calf has had difficulty bearing weight on the thoracic limbs for approximately 1 week. The calf appeared normal for the first 3 months of its life and is in excellent body condition. The calf spends a lot of time in sternal recumbency and has difficulty raising itself. The calf is bright and alert and propels itself along on its knees using the pelvic limbs (87).

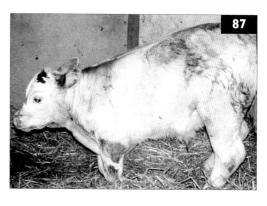

i. How do you determine the probable site of the neurological lesion?
ii. Where is the lesion?
iii. What lesion would you suspect? (Most likely first.)
iv. What ancillary tests could you undertake?
v. What is the prognosis?

88 You are presented with a 10-year-old Hereford-cross-Friesian suckler cow with an ocular lesion involving the right eye. The farmer has noticed a slight purulent unilateral ocular discharge and reddening of the lower eyelid for the past month or so. The lower eyelid margin of the right eye is hyperaemic and granular in appearance (88). Partial eversion of the lower eyelid reveals numerous irregular 3–5 mm reddened nodules. There is no involvement of the nictitans. The right submandibular lymph node is not enlarged.

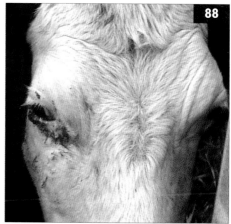

i. What conditions would you consider?
ii. What actions/treatments would you recommend?

87 i. A detailed neurological examination should be performed paying particular attention to the spinal reflex arcs. There are lower motor neuron signs to the thoracic limbs with reduced reflexes and flaccid paralysis, and upper motor neuron signs to pelvic limbs with increased reflexes and spastic paralysis.

ii. The lesion lies between C6 and T2.

iii. The most likely lesion is vertebral empyema, originating in one of the articular facets and extending to involve the vertebral body and vertebral canal causing cord compression. Despite the chronic nature of the empyema (several weeks to months), the calf may present with sudden onset of neurological signs. *Salmonella* serotypes, especially *S. dublin*, can cause such bone infections.

Other possible lesions include: vertebral body fracture (would cause sudden onset of neurological signs and pain associated with movement of the head, more commonly affects C4/C5); sarcocystis is a cause of recumbency in neonatal calves but not growing cattle; vitamin E/selenium deficiency (recumbency caused by white muscle disease presents as a bright, alert calf weak on all four legs).

iv. Further tests to identify a vertebral body lesion (bone lysis) are difficult even with excellent-quality radiographs. Myelography can be performed but is expensive and is not without risk. Lumbosacral CSF analysis is a useful indicator of an inflammatory lesion causing spinal cord compression, with an increase in protein from 0.3 g/L (0.03 g/dL) to >1.2 g/L (>0.12 g/dL).

v. Compressive spinal cord lesions, whether traumatic or inflammatory in origin, offer a grave prognosis.

88 i. The most likely conditions to consider include: ocular squamous cell carcinoma; trauma (foreign body) with secondary bacterial infection; infectious bovine keratoconjunctivitis. The clinical appearance, age, and breed of the cow are consistent with a diagnosis of ocular squamous cell carcinoma. The appearance suggests that the tumour is probably malignant.

ii. Enucleation and removal of the lower eyelid can be undertaken under xylazine sedation and a retrobulbar block using 2% lidocaine and NSAID pre-surgery. In this situation the farmer elects to cull the cow because she is 10 years old and coming to the end of her productive life in the herd. Surgery would involve stitching the eyelids closed, then making an elliptical incision near the orbit rim and blunt disection between the eye and socket. The optic stump is grasped with artery forceps but ligation is very difficult; the stump is then cut. The socket is packed with sterile swabs and the eyelids are sutured together. The packing is removed after 3–4 days. Surprisingly, there are few complications.

89 A Holstein heifer, which calved 2 months ago, presents with marked lameness (9/10) of the right pelvic limb with muscle atrophy over the affected limb, and general body condition loss. The lateral claw is slightly swollen around the bulb of the heel and the heifer holds the leg abducted with the weight borne by the medial claw. There is considerable new horn production and consequent bruising of the sole (**89a**).

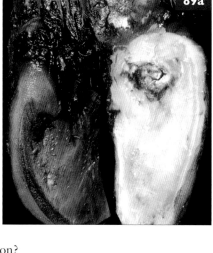

i. What conditions would you consider? (Most likely first.)
ii. What action would you take?
iii. What are the potential consequences?
iv. What factors contribute to this condition?
v. How could the prevalence of this problem be reduced?

90 A 5-year-old dairy cow, due to calve in 6 weeks, presents with 4 weeks' history of increasing abdominal distension since drying off. The cow is bright and alert, and eating well. The abdomen is markedly distended ventrally on both sides (**90**). The rectal temperature is normal. The force and rate of rumen contractions is normal (one cycle every 40 s).

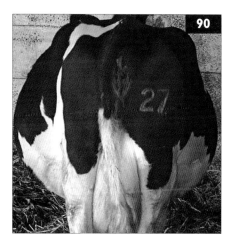

i. What conditions would you consider? (Most likely first.)
ii. How could you confirm your diagnosis?
iii. What actions/treatments would you recommend?

89 i. The most likely conditions to consider include: sole ulcer; septic pedal arthritis; white line abscess extending to coronary band; digital dermatitis; interdigital necrobacillosis.

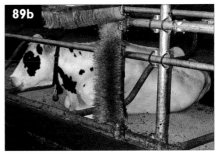

ii. Careful paring reveals a sole ulcer. There is no swelling at the coronary band on the abaxial aspect of the hoof wall which would suggest deep sepsis. The exuberant granulation tissue is excised level with the sole and a pressure bandage applied. A wooden block is glued to the sound claw.

iii. Potential consequences of sole ulcer include infection that can gain entry into the navicular bursa, distal interphalangeal (coffin) joint causing swelling at the coronary band, and deep flexor tendon sheath with swelling extending to the mid-metatarsal region. Rupture of the deep digital flexor tendon results in unopposed pull of the extensor tendon on the third phalanx with the toe 'knocked up'. The possibility of deep infection could be investigated by radiography or arthrocentesis. An alternative technique is to inject sterile saline into the distal interphalangeal joint and observe whether it appears at the site of the sole ulcer.

iv. Factors which contribute to this condition include poor leg and foot conformation and altered weightbearing due to abnormal horn growth. Compression of the solear corium between the horn of the sole and the caudal aspect of P3 accounts for the characteristic position. Poorly designed uncomfortable cubicles, insufficient bedding material, and high-concentrate/low-roughage rations are also important factors.

v. The disease prevalence could be reduced by providing an adequate number of Dutch comfort cubicles (**89b**) or loose housing on straw bedding, and foot trimming every 6 months.

90 i. The most likely conditions to consider include: twin pregnancy; high-fibre diet/low protein intake during the dry period; vagus indigestion; hydrops allantois (hydrallantois). This presentation is consistent with a twin pregnancy.

ii. There is no confirmatory test at this stage of gestation for twins. Hydrops allantois develops rapidly (over several days) during the 6th/7th month of gestation.

iii. There should be free access to the diet, especially any concentrates. BCS should be monitored closely. If there is concern over body condition loss, 3-OH butyrate concentration should be measured (<0.6 mmol/L (<6.0 mg/dL) guideline). The cow should be supervised closely for first-stage labour as dystocia is common in twin pregnancies. The cow calved twin calves unaided at day 278 of gestation (several days earlier than expected but this is not unusual).

91 A 2-month-old Holstein heifer calf presents with poor appetite and low weight gain since birth (**91a**). The calf is dull and lethargic. The rectal temperature is normal (38.4°C (101.1°F)). The ocular and oral mucous membranes are pink. The heart rate is 90 beats per minute. Auscultation of the chest reveals a harsh pansystolic murmur in the tricuspid valve area. The murmur is louder on the right than the left side. A

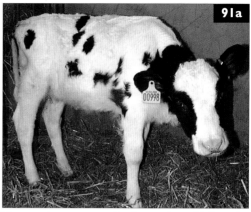

palpable cardiac thrill is present. The respiratory rate is elevated to 44 breaths per minute with a slight abdominal component.
i. Which conditions would you consider?
ii. What is the prognosis?

92 In early summer you are presented with an 8-year-old Normandy-cross beef suckler cow which calved 6 months ago. The cow has been at pasture for 1 week with a group of autumn-calving cows receiving no supplementary feeding. The cow was found separated from other cows, frothing at the mouth, and unsteady. The cow had been walked approximately 400 m

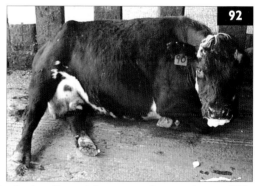

into the cattle shed whereupon she had collapsed into sternal recumbency (**92**). Visual assessment indicates that there is no bloat. The cow appears hyperaesthetic and makes rapid jerking movements with her head. The cow makes a number of attempts to stand. Eventually the cow gains her feet but appears ataxic with a very stilted gait. The cow is aggressive and makes a lunge at you tossing her head vigorously.
i. What conditions would you consider?
ii. What treatments would you administer?
iii. How could this condition be prevented?

91 i. The most likely conditions to consider include: ventricular septal defect; patent ductus arteriosus; tetralogy of Fallot.

ii. The prognosis is hopeless and the calf was euthanased for welfare reasons. Postmortem examination confirmed the presence of a moderate defect located high in the septum separating the ventricles just ventral to the aortic valve in the left ventricle (91b). No other cardiac defects were present.

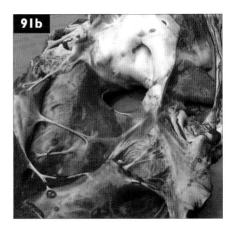

92 i. The most likely conditions to consider include: hypomagnesaemia; listeriosis; bovine spongiform encephalopathy; lead poisoning; malignant catarrhal fever; rabies.

A diagnosis of hypomagnesaemia is based upon the clinical findings and history of recent turnout to pasture. The cows are receiving no supplementary magnesium. There is no bloat to indicate an oesophageal foreign body.

ii. The cow is too aggressive and unsteady to walk to the cattle stocks. The cow is jammed behind a gate and sedated with 6 mL of 20% pentobarbital solution injected intravenously into the tail vein (note that this preparation is not licensed for use in cattle in many countries but alternative sedatives such as xylazine and diazepam do not work nearly so well). Within minutes the cow is more relaxed and no longer aggressive.

The cow can now be safely haltered and approximately 50 mL of 25% magnesium sulphate solution is added to 400 mL of 40% calcium borogluconate and the mixture given very slowly by intravenous injection over approximately 15 minutes. The remainder of the 400 mL bottle of 25% magnesium sulphate solution is given immediately behind the left shoulder at two divided sites to aid absorption. The cow appears much less excitable and the frothy salivation is less pronounced. The cow is normal within 6 hr and returns to pasture the following day.

iii. Prevention includes feeding 2 kg of high-magnesium cobs per cow per day for several weeks following turnout to pasture in the spring. Barley straw should also be available to the cows.

93 A 5-day-old Charolais-cross beef calf has been dull and unwilling to suckle from the cow for the past 6 hr. The rectal temperature is 39.2°C (102.6°F). The calf is depressed and stands with a wide-based stance with the neck extended (93a). The menace response is reduced and there is marked episcleral congestion and dorsomedial strabismus. The respiratory rate is increased at 60 breaths per minute. The umbilicus had been treated with strong iodine solution and appears normal. There is no evidence of diarrhoea. The lymph nodes are not enlarged.

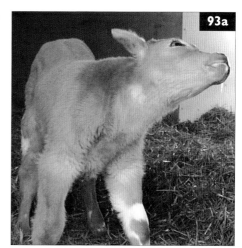

i. What conditions would you consider?
ii. How could you confirm your diagnosis?
iii. What is the likely cause?
iv. What treatment(s) would you administer?
v. What is the prognosis for this calf?

94 In early autumn you are presented with an 18-month-old beef heifer which is much smaller than other bulling heifers in the group (220 kg versus 370 kg) (94). The heifers are unvaccinated and purchased from numerous sources. A bull has been with the group for 4 months. Recently, the heifer has developed diarrhoea but some other heifers in the group are also affected. Clinical exam-

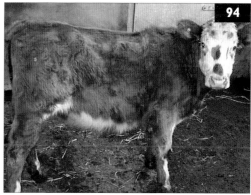

ination reveals pyrexia (39.1°C (102.4°F)), slight mucopurulent ocular and nasal discharges, and peripheral lymphadenopathy.
i. What conditions would you consider? (Most likely first.)
ii. What tests would you undertake?
iii. What other clinical problems could be expected?

93, 94: Answers

93 i. The most likely conditions to consider include: bacterial meningoencephalitis; septicaemia.

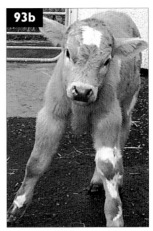

ii. Diagnosis of meningoencephalitis follows lumbar CSF collection under local anaesthesia using a 20-gauge 25 mm hypodermic needle. The sample is turbid, caused by the influx of white cells, and has a frothy appearance after sample agitation due to the increased protein concentration. Laboratory analysis reveals a total protein concentration of 1.1 g/L (0.11 g/dL) (normal <0.3 g/L, <0.03 g/dL) with a white cell concentration of 1.6×10^9/L (1.6×10^3/µL) (normal $<0.012 \times 10^9$/L, $<0.012 \times 10^3$/µL), comprised almost entirely of neutrophils (neutrophilic pleocytosis). The total plasma protein of 48 g/L (4.8 g/dL) indicates failure of passive antibody transfer (normal value for calves that have sucked colostrum >65 g/L, <6.5 g/dL).

iii. *Escherichia coli*, *Pasteurella* spp., *Staphylococcus pyogenes*, and *Arcanobacterium pyogenes* have been isolated from clinical cases of meningoencephalitis. *E. coli* is the most common isolate from septicaemic calves.

iv. The calf was treated with high doses of intravenous trimethoprim/sulphonamide and soluble corticosteroid (dexamethasone at 1.0 mg/kg).

v. The calf improved over the next 24 hr (**93b**).

94 i. The most likely conditions to consider include: persistent infection with BVD virus; type I ostertigiasis; chronic suppurative pneumonia; IBR; salmonellosis; 'recovered' case of malignant catarrhal fever.

ii. A blood sample result was BVD virus antibody negative, antigen positive. The faecal culture was negative for *Salmonella* and the faecal worm egg count was low at 200 strongyle epg (probably *Ostertagia* spp.). Lithium heparin blood samples could be collected from all the remaining heifers in the group to identify other heifers persistently infected with BVD virus, although transient infection could interfere with interpretation.

iii. Potential problems could include a poor pregnancy rate in seronegative heifers due to embryonic/early fetal death if infected by BVD virus. *In utero* infection of the developing fetus in a seronegative heifer between 45 and 135 days results in the birth of a persistently infected calf with cerebellar hypoplasia a common manifestation of late fetal infection. Transient infertility of the bull could result after virus infection if he was seronegative. Abortions can be expected at 4–7 months of gestation.

95 With regard to the beef heifer in case **94**, how could this scenario have been prevented?

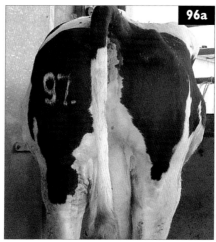

96 A 6-year-old beef cow presents with 10 days' history of inappetance and severe weight loss. The cow was treated by the farmer for interdigital necrobacillosis with long-acting oxytetracycline injection 2 weeks ago. The rectal temperature is normal (38.6°C (101.5°F)). The cow is slow when walking and there is slight effusion of the left hind fetlock joint and both hock joints. There is a large hot and painful (>25 cm diameter) swelling on the lateral aspect of both hindlegs immediately proximal to the stifle joints (**96a**).

Routine haematological examination reveals mild anaemia (total red blood cell count 4.8 10^{12}/L (4.8 × 10^{6}/µL), normal range 5–9 × 10^{12}/L (5–9 × 10^{6}/µL); haemoglobin 76 g/L (7.6 g/dL), normal range 80–140 g/L (8–14 g/dL)). There is a slight leucocytosis (11.2 × 10^{9}/L, 11.2 × 10^{3}/µL), resulting from a marginal neutrophilia. There are significant changes in the serum albumin and globulin concentrations (16.8 g/L (1.68 g/dL) and 66.3 g/L (6.63 g/dL), normal range >30g/L (>3 g/dL) and 35–45 g/L (3.5–4.5 g/dL), respectively).

i. What conditions would you consider? (Most likely first.)
ii. How could you confirm your provisional diagnosis?
iii. What treatment would you recommend?
iv. What is the prognosis?

95 Prevention of disease could involve establishment and maintenance of a BVD-/MD-free herd. A vaccination programme of all breeding cattle would appear to be the safest option where doubts exist over biosecurity.

96 i. The most likely conditions to consider include: cellulitis/large abscesses; haematomata; bacterial endocarditis; multiple joint effusions associated with chronic bacterial infection; polyarthritis.

ii. Real-time B-mode examination of the right side swelling with a 5 MHz sector scanner revealed an anechoic area with a hyperechoic lattice-work appearance extending for 12 cm, consistent with an organized haematoma or cellulitis (96b). The left swelling appeared anechoic with multiple hyperechoic dots consistent with a deep-seated abscess/cellulitis. Needle aspiration of the swellings yielded red–brown, foul-smelling fluid consistent with infected haematomata/cellulitis.

iii. Treatment with 44,000 IU/kg procaine penicillin administered intramusculary twice daily was commenced and dexamethasone was given intravenously once only. The cow was less lame and her appetite was increased and this improvement continued for approximately 6 days after which the cow deteriorated to her condition at first presentation. There was no significant improvement in the clinical presentation over the next 5 days, therefore the cow was euthanased for welfare reasons.

iv. Postmortem examination revealed extensive deep-seated cellulitis lesions with muscle necrosis consistent with iatrogenic introduction of infection with the needle/injection solution rather than infected haematomas.

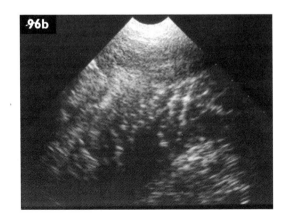

97 You are called to a small 4-day-old Limousin-cross heifer calf from a dairy herd. The calf has been dull and unwilling to suck since early morning. The calf has deteriorated rapidly and is very depressed and presents in sternal recumbency (97), being unable to stand even when assisted to its feet. The calf has sunken eyes and the skin tent is extended to 4 s. The rectal temperature is 37.2°C (99.0°F). The menace response is reduced but this is

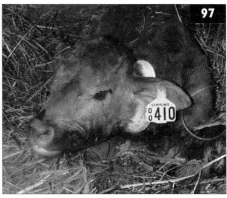

difficult to judge because the calf is so depressed. There is marked episcleral congestion. The mucous membranes are congested. The respiratory rate is increased at 40 breaths per minute. The abdomen is shrunken and there is little content in the abomasum/intestines, despite administration of 2 L of oral rehydration solution by oesophageal feeder 4 hr earlier. There is slight thickening of the umbilical remnant which is covered by an infected scab. There is recent evidence of diarrhoea with staining of the tail and perineum. The farmer states that there was no evidence of diarrhoea earlier this morning. The joints and carcass lymph nodes are not enlarged. The farmer is unsure whether the calf sucked colostrum within the first 6 hr after birth.
i. What conditions would you consider?
ii. What treatment(s) would you administer?
iii. What is the prognosis for this calf?

98 You are called to a 4-year-old Limousin-cross-Friesian cow to assist delivery of a calf in posterior presentation with bilateral hip flexion (breech presentation) (98). The cow is in sternal recumbency with the calf's pelvis firmly lodged within the maternal pelvis. The cow shows forceful abdominal contractions.
i. How will you deliver this calf?
ii. What risks are associated with this presentation?

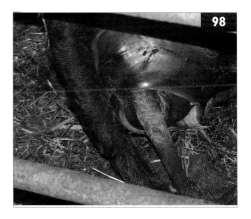

97 i. The most likely conditions to consider include: septicaemia associated with failure of passive antibody transfer; bacterial meningoencephalitis; enterotoxigenic *Escherichia coli*; dehydration and acidosis associated with diarrhoea.

Determination of total plasma protein concentration using a refractometer reveals a concentration of 42 g/L (4.2 g/dL) consistent with failure of passive transfer (normal >65 g/L, >6.5 g/dL). Inspection of lumbar CSF collected under local anaesthesia using a 20-gauge 25 mm hypodermic needle reveals a normal, clear, and colourless sample.

ii. The calf was treated with trimethoprim/sulphonamide given intravenously. Ketoprofen (a NSAID) was also injected intravenously. The calf was catheterized and 3 L of isotonic saline infused over 6 hr (approximately 1.5 L was infused over the first 30 minutes).

iii. The prognosis for septicaemia in neonatal calves is guarded. This calf appeared much brighter after 30 minutes but died approximately 12 hr after veterinary examination. Failure of passive antibody transfer, as in this case, and a heavily contaminated environment predispose neonates to septicaemia. The farmer was advised that all newborn calves must receive colostrum equivalent to 7% of their bodyweight within the first 6 hr of life.

98 i. The cow is first ushered into cattle stocks and 5 mL of 2% lidocaine injected extradurally at the sacrococcygeal site to reduce the forceful abdominal contractions. Flunixin meglumine is injected intravenously for pain relief. Five minutes after the low extradural block, the calf's tailhead is slowly repelled to the level of the cow's pelvic inlet. Commencing distally, one calf's foot is cupped in a hand and the fetlock joint fully flexed. As the calf's hindfoot is drawn toward the maternal pelvis, the hock and stifle joints are fully flexed. Correction now involves extending each hip joint in turn while the distal limb joints (stifle, hock, and fetlock joints) remain fully flexed. Further gentle repulsion of the calf may be necessary at this stage. In this manner a breech presentation is converted to a posterior presentation. To proceed safely with attempted delivery by traction the calf's hindlegs must protrude a hand's breadth beyond the hocks after a maximum period of 10 minutes' traction by two people. The decision must be reconsidered if greater traction is necessary to pull the calf to this stage because there is the risk of serious trauma to both the cow and calf.

ii. Risks associated with delivery include: (1) Calf – rib fractures at the costochondral junction if it is a large calf and excessive traction is applied; premature rupture of the umbilical vessels if the umbilicus has become hooked around one hindleg while correcting the hip flexion. (2) Dam – uterine rupture during retropulsion of the calf or correction of the hip flexion; vaginal tear during delivery causing haemorrhage.

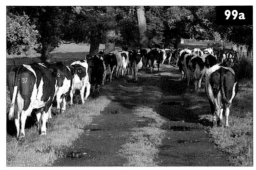

99 Arriving on a farm at milking time in June you observe the milking herd snaking its way along a farm track to the milking parlour (**99a**).
i. Is this farm track suitable for cattle?
ii. What conditions could result from these underfoot conditions? (Most likely first.)
iii. What action should be taken?

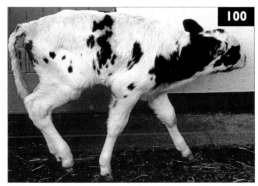

100 A Holstein calf in anterior presentation was delivered by a farmer using a calving aid but considerable force was necessary when the calf became hip-locked. For the first 2 weeks the calf was only able bear weight on its thoracic limbs and was often observed dog-sitting. Now, 3 weeks old, the calf is able to bear weight on the right hindleg (**100**).
i. What conditions would you consider? (Most likely first.)
ii. How could this problem have been avoided?
iii. What is the prognosis for this calf?
iv. What are the other common consequences of such dystocia?

99, 100: Answers

99 i. This farm track is not suitable for cattle. Note that along some parts of the track the cows follow the single-file track free of large sharp stones (98b).

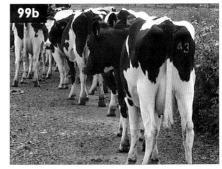

ii. The most likely conditions that could result from these underfoot conditions include: stone becomes lodged in the interdigital space predisposing to interdigital necrobacillosis; penetration of the sole by a sharp stone with abscess formation; white line separation/impacted material causing white line abscess; repeated trauma causing bruising of the sole which may lead to sole ulcer.

iii. Immediate action would include sweeping the track free of large sharp stones. The track should be resurfaced with the correct material.

100 i. The most likely conditions to consider include: femoral nerve paralysis; femoral fracture(s) particularly through the proximal epiphysis; dislocated hip; pelvic fracture; spinal cord trauma; congenital sarcocystosis.

Excessive traction of oversized calves in anterior longitudinal presentation causes femoral nerve trauma. The femoral nerve supplies the quadriceps femoris muscle and injury results in rapid and severe atrophy, and the inability to extend the stifle joint and bear weight on that leg. Bilateral femoral paralysis results in the inability to stand and should be differentiated from a spinal lesion caudal to T2. Fractures of long bones following dystocia are rare but can occur. Such fractures can be detected by careful clinical examination and radiography.

ii. Two people pulling a calf presented in anterior longitudinal presentation should be able to extend both foreleg fetlock joints one hand's breadth beyond the cow's vulva (indicates extension of the calf's elbows into the pelvis) within 10 minutes. Any greater traction to achieve such progress forewarns of possible hip-lock and its consequences (this case). Rotation of the calf by 45° into a diagonal orientation to align the widest dimension of the calf's hips with the widest dimension of the maternal pelvis may assist delivery in some cases. This problem should have been avoided by caesarean operation.

iii. The prognosis for bilateral femoral nerve paralysis is frequently hopeless despite intensive nursing and supportive care. Full recovery for unilateral femoral nerve trauma may take up to 9 months.

iv. Other common consequences of such dystocia include septicaemia and infections such as meningitis, polyarthritis, hypopyon, and omphlophlebitis, due to delay/failure of passive antibody transfer.

101 A 10-day-old bucket-fed calf presents with a large (4 cm diameter) swelling of the right cheek (**101**). Oral examination reveals that the lesion extends through the buccal mucosa into the cheek muscles. The right submandibular lymph node is enlarged. The calf is bright and alert and drinking well. The rectal temperature is 39.1°C (102.4°F). The mucous membranes are normal. Examination of the mouth reveals a large diphtheritic lesion with a necrotic centre in the left cheek extending into the cheek muscles.

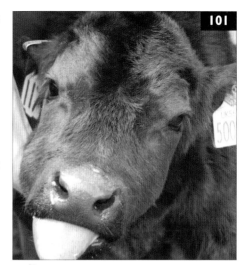

i. What conditions would you consider?
ii. What treatments would you recommend?
iii. Are there any sequelae?
iv. What control measures would you recommend?

102 You are presented with a 5-year-old Holstein cow 3 days after assisted delivery of live twins. The cow has a daily milk yield of only 12 L. On clinical examination the cow is dull and depressed, inappetant, with a poor milk yield. The cow is febrile with a rectal temperature of 40.2°C (104.4°F). The cow has diarrhoea but there is no evidence of blood or mucosal casts in the faeces. The mucous membranes are congested. The vulva is

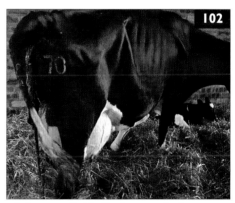

slightly swollen with evidence of a red–brown fluid discharge. At least one placenta is retained (**102**).

i. What is your diagnosis?
ii. What treatments would you consider?
iii. What are the possible consequences?
iv. What factors are believed to contribute to retained placenta?

101 i. The most likely conditions to consider include: calf diphtheria; foreign body/trauma; actinobacillosis.

ii. The organism most commonly isolated from cases of calf diphtheria is *Fusobacterium necrophorum*. The commonly used antibiotics include procaine penicillin, trimethoprim/sulphonamide, and amoxicillin/clavulanic acid (always use the simplest, and cheapest, antibiotic, i.e. procaine penicillin). Intramuscular penicillin was injected intramuscularly at 44,000 IU/kg once daily for 10 consecutive days. The following day the cheek swelling was considerably reduced. Supportive care during convalescence, e.g. soft feed, can be beneficial.

iii. Sequelae include infection extending to involve the larynx (necrotic laryngitis, laryngeal necrobacillosis) and inhalation of infected material can result in pneumonia with characteristic large pleural abscesses, but these events are uncommon.

iv. Prevention through good husbandry controls this disease. Outbreaks of calf diphtheria occur under unhygienic conditions with transmission between animals via dirty milk buckets. The importance of strict hygiene and thorough cleaning and disinfection of the milk buckets between feeds must be emphasized. Occasionally, outbreaks can occur on beef farms where infection is transmitted by dirty oesophageal feeders used to administer colostrum and oral rehydration solutions to calves.

102 i. The most likely conditions to consider include: metritis; metritis and left-displaced abomasum; salmonellosis; endotoxaemia/toxaemia; ruptured uterus and associated peritonitis.

ii. Treatment includes intravenous oxytetracycline and flunixin meglumine, then intramucular oxytetracycline for the following 2 days. There is debate regarding the amount of time and effort that should be taken to remove placenta(e) retained after the third day postpartum. Often a knot of placenta is retained by the contracted cervix and can be removed by gentle traction. Separation of individual placentomes is not recommended due to the endometrial damage that results. As a general rule if the placenta(e) are still attached on the third day postpartum apply slight traction to that portion of the placenta(e) protruding through the cervix and the placenta(e) should come away easily. If the placenta(e) tears apart, leave for another 2 days and try again.

iii. Chronic endometritis is a likely sequel to acute metritis and the cow should be presented 14–28 days after calving. The use of intrauterine antibiotic infusions is widely practised at that time or injection with a prostaglandin preparation.

iv. Factors contributing to retained fetal membranes and metritis include twins, induced parturition, abortion, hypocalcaemia, interference/unskilled assistance during dystocia correction, and poor hygiene in the calving accommodation.

103 You are presented with a 6-year-old pedigree Simmental cow 2 weeks after a 'difficult calving' (two calves presented simultaneously) corrected by the farmer. The cow was normal for the first few days but thereafter she has had a poor appetite and both calves are now being reared artificially due to the cow's poor milk yield. The cow has received two 5-day courses of antibiotics (amoxicillin plus clavulanic acid, then oxytetracy-

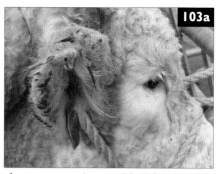

cline) but with little improvement. The rectal temperature is now 38.4°C (101.1°F). The cow has a painful facial expression (103a) and a slightly arched back. The mucous membranes appear pale and the cow is about 5–7% dehydrated. The heart rate is 96 beats per minute. The abdomen appears distended contrasting with the reduced appetite. The rumen contractions are reduced with only one cycle per 2 minutes. There are scant firm faeces in the rectum. The uterus extends over the pelvic brim.

i. What conditions would you consider?
ii. Which further tests could be undertaken on the farm?
iii. What actions/treatments would you recommend?
iv. What prevention measures would you recommend?

104 You are asked to 'cleanse' a 4-year-old Limousin-cross beef cow which calved 3 days previously (104). The cow had an assisted calving as a consequence of absolute fetal oversize. The cow is bright and alert, and is eating well. The rectal temperature is marginally elevated (39.0°C (102.2°F)). There are several large diphtheritic lesions immediately within the vagina as a consequence of the dystocia.

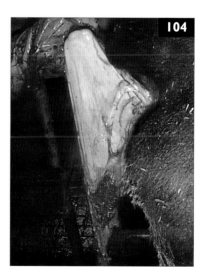

i. What would you do?
ii. Is removing retained fetal membranes around day 3 a good idea?
iii. What advice would you offer?

111

103 i. The most likely conditions to consider include: diffuse septic peritonitis (associated with a uterine tear?); traumatic reticulitis; septic metritis; abdominal catastrophe – abomasal volvulus, intestinal torsion, proximal duodenal obstruction.

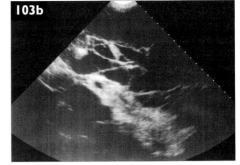

ii. Ultrasonography of the lower right flank reveals an extensive fibrinous matrix extending beyond the 20 cm depth of a 5 MHz sector scanner (**103b**). With such findings, abdominocentesis is not necessary to confirm the severe extensive (septic) peritonitis.

iii. Diffuse septic peritonitis does not respond to antibiotic therapy as evidenced by the previous antibiotic therapy administered by the farmer. Peritoneal cavity lavage using large quantities of very dilute povidone–iodine solution has been reported to be successful in a limited number of early cases of peritonitis but not this case. The cow was euthanased for welfare reasons and the extent of the peritonitis was revealed via a right flank incision on the farm. It was not possible to undertake a full necropsy on farm, therefore the cause could not be conclusively proven but a uterine tear is the probable cause.

iv. Veterinary assistance at calving would have prevented this unfortunate outcome.

104 i. The cow is not ill and there is no evidence of toxic metritis. A gloved hand is gently inserted up to the cervix and the fetal membranes grasped and gentle traction applied. If the fetal membranes are retained only by the contracted cervix they will drop out within 2 minutes.

ii. Frequently, the fetal membranes are retained only by the contracted cervix and readily fall out with minimal traction. If this is not successful, the farmer is instructed to leave the cow another 2 or 3 days before attempting this procedure again. Passing through the cervix and peeling the fetal membranes from every caruncle is generally not recommended as the resultant trauma may increase toxin absorption across the uterine wall. There are few studies on the effects of endometritis on the subsequent fertility performance of beef cows. The farmer was advised that this cow should be treated with prostaglandin F2 alpha at around 21 days postpartum.

iii. Attention should be paid to reducing the incidence of predisposing factors, most commonly dystocia from absolute fetal oversize, by bull selection using estimated transmitting ability values. Twinning is also a common cause of retained fetal membranes in beef cows but there is no obvious control.

105 A 4-year-old Limousin-cross beef cow presents with a large swelling extending from immediately cranial to the udder to the xiphisternum and halfway up the abdominal wall which pits readily under digital pressure (105a). The swelling was first noted 4 days ago. The cow calved 5 months previously. The cow is bright and alert with a BCS of 2.5 (scale 1–5). The cow appears stiff on

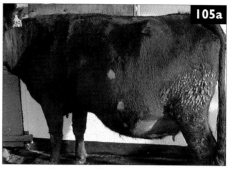

the left hindleg and has difficulty protracting the leg. The rectal temperature is normal (38.6°C (101.5°F)). The ocular and oral mucous membranes are pale. The heart rate is 82 beats per minute, and respiratory rate 22 breaths per minute.
i. What conditions would you consider?
ii. How could you confirm your provisional diagnosis?
iii. What treatment would you recommend?
iv. What is the prognosis?

106 A 6-year-old Limousin beef cow presents with 2 weeks' history of poor appetite and weight loss (106). The cow calved 2 months ago. The rectal temperature is marginally elevated (39.2°C (102.6°F)). The ocular and oral mucous membranes are slightly pale. The heart rate is 70 beats per minute. The respiratory rate is 24 breaths per minute with no abnormal sounds detected on auscultation of the chest. The ruminal contractions

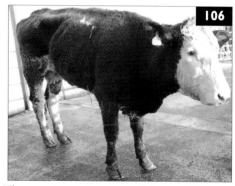

are reduced in strength and frequency. The cow is passing normal faeces. The cow makes frequent attempts to urinate but only a small amount of urine is voided which contains some flecks of blood and a small amount of pus. The cow resents rectal palpation, which reveals thickened bladder wall and ureters.
i. What conditions would you consider? (Most likely first.)
ii. How could you confirm your provisional diagnosis?
iii. What is the prognosis?
iv. What treatment would you recommend?

105 i. The most likely conditions to consider include: massive haematoma (rupture of the left pudendal artery?); abscess/cellulitis; ruptured prepubic tendon; ascites.

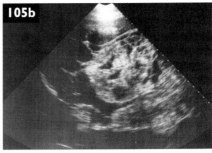

ii. Real-time B-mode ultrasonographic examination of the swelling is undertaken with a 5 MHz sector scanner. The swelling extends for at least 20 cm (depth of 5 MHz ultrasound scanner field). There are large pockets of fluid (anechoic areas) within a matrix typical of an organizing haematoma (hyperechoic lines) (105b). The swelling did not have the sonographic appearance of an abscess ('snowstorm' appearance).

Routine haematological examination revealed a regenerative anaemia (total red blood cell count 2.8×10^{12}/L (2.8×10^6/µL) with an occasional normoblast, normal range $5–9 \times 10^{12}$/L ($5–9 \times 10^6$/µL); haemoglobin 56 g/L (5.6 g/dL), normal range 80–140 g/L (8–14 g/dL)). The total white blood cell count and differential counts were within normal ranges. There were no significant changes in the serum albumin and globulin concentrations (32.8 g/L (3.28 g/dL) and 46.3 g/L (4.63 g/dL), respectively). No attempt was made to tap the swelling.

iii. There is no specific treatment for this haematoma.

iv. The prognosis is good provided that the haemotoma does not become infected.

106 i. The most likely conditions to consider include: cystitis/pyelonephritis; bladder tumour; chronic endometritis; Johne's disease; chronic peritonitis.

ii. Urinalysis reveals a strong positive result for protein, blood, and white blood cells, consistent with cystitis/pyelonephritis. A direct smear of midstream urine sediment yields Gram-positive rods. The BUN concentration is 14.9 mmol/L (41.7 mg/dL) (normal range 2–6 mmol/L, 5.6–16.8 mg/dL). There is a slight leucocytosis (10.4×10^9/L, 10.4×10^3/µL), resulting from a marginal neutrophilia. There is a marked hypoalbuminaemia and elevated globulin concentration (18.8 g/L (1.9 g/dL) and 61.3 g/L (6.1 g/dL), respectively), consistent with chronic bacterial infection. Bacteriological culture of a urine sample yields a pure growth of *Corynebacterium renale*.

Transrectal ultrasonography using a linear scanner typically reveals a markedly thickened bladder wall (>1 cm).

iii. The prognosis for pyelonephritis is very poor, despite prolonged antibiotic therapy, due to the extent of kidney destruction; some improvements can be made in the short-term which may allow slaughter.

iv. Penicillin is excreted in the urine and is very effective against *C. renale*. Treatment should be administered intramusculary once daily for 3–6 weeks.

107 The sonogram (107a) was obtained with a 5.0 MHz sector transducer, connected to a real-time, B-mode ultrasound machine, placed in the lower right sublumbar fossa of a 3-year-old bull. The bull has not eaten for 3 days and has passed only thick mucus. Despite this period of inappetance the bull has obvious abdominal distension. There are no rumen con-

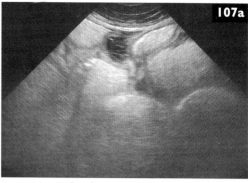

tractions. There is marked dehydration, estimated to be 5–7% (PCV 0.45 L/L). The rectal temperature is 39.1°C (102.4°F). The heart rate is 110 beats per minute.

i. Describe the important sonographic findings.
ii. What further tests might you undertake?
iii. What causes would you consider? (Most likely first.)
iv. How could you confirm your diagnosis?
v. What is the prognosis?

108 A beef cow has been unable to bear weight on the right foreleg since colliding with a fence during handling through the cattle stocks 2 weeks ago. The rectal temperature is 38.5°C (101.3°F). There is a loss of muscle over the scapula with a prominent spine. There is a dropped elbow, flexion of the distal limb joints, and scuffing of the hooves as the leg is moved forward (108). The foot is knuckled over at rest. The right

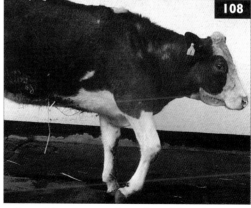

prescapular lymph node is not swollen. Muscle tone is reduced but it proves difficult to test the reflex arcs.

i. What conditions would you consider? (Most likely first.)
ii. What treatment(s) would you administer?
iii. What is the prognosis for this cow?

107, 108: Answers

107 i. Ultrasonographic examination reveals massive fluid distension of loops of small intestine (up to 6–8 cm) with small pockets of fluid containing fibrin tags which bridge adjacent loops.

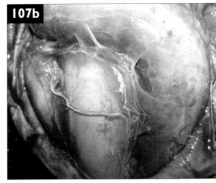

ii. Rectal examination would confirm the extent of small intestine distension. Ultrasound-guided abdominocentesis would establish whether the fluid was a transudate or inflammatory exudate. A protein concentration >30 g/L (>3.0 g/dL) indicates an inflammatory exudate.

iii. The most likely conditions to consider include: diffuse fibrinous peritonitis; small intestine volvulus; intussusception; ileus.

iv. The diagnosis could be confirmed after right flank laporotomy. Surgery could be performed under paravertebral anaesthesia undertaken after intravenous flunixin and hypertonic saline infusion (7.2%; 5 mL/kg in 5–7 minutes) followed by isotonic saline to stabilize the bull for standing surgery. Surgery would be ill advised in this case due to the poor prognosis.

v. The prognosis is hopeless, particularly in view of the peritonitis, and the bull should be euthanased for welfare reasons. A heart rate above 100 beats per minutes affords a poor prognosis. The serum chloride concentration was 74 mmol/L (74 mEq/L); <80 mmol/L (<80 mEq/L) indicates a poor prognosis. Determination of anion gap ($Na^+ + K^+ - Cl^-$) may be more accurate than chloride alone. Necropsy revealed diffuse fibrinous peritonitis. Rupture of the small intestine occurred despite careful handling at necropsy (107b). Ultrasonographic examination of peritonitis cases often fails to reveal the true extent and severity of the condition because of the limited depth of field of the probe compared to the abdominal size.

108 i. The most likely conditions to consider include: radial nerve paralysis following trauma in the mid/distal humeral region; trauma or infection of the shoulder/elbow joints; severe foot lesion (foot abscess, septic pedal arthritis).

ii. Clinical examination failed to reveal any skeletal abnormality and a provisional diagnosis of radial nerve paralysis was reached. The cow was isolated with her calf in a small paddock.

iii. The cow showed signs of improvement after 1 month and was fully recovered after 4 months.

109 A 3-year-old Holstein cow presents with 2 weeks' history of poor milk yield, reduced appetite, marked weight loss, and stiffness. The cow is dull and depressed with a painful expression and stands with a roached back and abducts the elbows (**109a**). The rectal temperature is normal (39.1°C (102.4°F)). There is effusion of both hock joints and all four fetlock joints. The heart rate is 90 beats per minute with a systolic murmur audible on the left

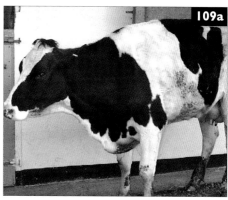

side over the mitral valve area. The respiratory rate is 24 breaths per minute.
i. Which conditions would you consider? (Most likely first.)
ii. What treatment would you recommend?
iii. What is the prognosis?

110 You are presented with a depressed Hereford-cross-Friesian heifer, first noticed to be dull and disoriented 4 days ago. The heifer is easily haltered and restrained. The rectal temperature is 39.2°C (102.6°F). There is an obvious head tilt to the left. The left upper eyelid and left ear are drooped and there is lack of tone in the facial muscles on the left side causing deviation of the muzzle to the right side (**110**). There is profuse salivation and the heifer has difficulty swallowing; there is a large amount of silage material firmly impacted in the left cheek.

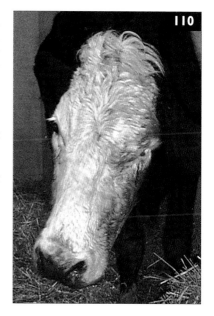

i. What conditions would you consider? (Most likely first.)
ii. What laboratory tests could be undertaken to confirm your provisional diagnosis?
iii. What treatment would you administer?
iv. What is the prognosis?

109 i. The most likely conditions to consider include: bacterial endocarditis; joint effusions associated with a chronic suppurative focus; septic polyarthritis; myocarditis; chronic suppurative pulmonary disease.

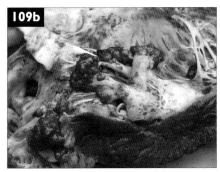

ii. The organisms isolated, often streptococci, are sensitive to penicillin. In this case, treatment with 44,000 IU/kg procaine penicillin administered daily was commenced and a single injection of dexamethasone given intramuscularly. The cow's appetite and milk yield increased but this improvement lasted approximately 1 week after which time the cow deteriorated to the condition at first presentation. The cow was euthanased for welfare reasons.

iii. The prognosis for bacterial endocarditis is poor due to the long-standing physical nature of the vegetative heart lesion, spread of septic emboli to other organs, and secondary changes in other organs due to chronic venous congestion. At necropsy a large vegetative lesion was present on the mitral valve (109b).

110 i. The most likely conditions to consider include: unilateral brainstem lesion – listeriosis; peripheral vestibular lesion; brain abscess; bovine spongiform encephalopathy; botulism.

ii. Analysis of lumbar CSF, collected from the standing animal under local anaesthesia using an 18-gauge 10 cm spinal needle (400–600 kg cattle), reveals an elevated CSF protein concentration of 1.4 g/L (0.14 g/dL) (normal <0.3 g/L, <0.03 g/dL), and a mild increase in white cell concentration (pleocytosis) comprised mainly of large mononuclear cells. Culture of CSF is unrewarding in listeriosis.

iii. Recovery of cattle from listerial encephalitis demands early detection of illness by the farmer, and aggressive antibiotic treatment. *Listeria monocytogenes* is susceptible to various antibiotics including penicillin, ceftiofur, erythromycin, and trimethoprim/sulphonamide. The initial daily dose of procaine penicillin is 200,000 IU/kg with emphasis on the maximum dose of penicillin costs will permit rather than worry about the duration of daily penicillin injections thereafter. A single intravenous injection of 1.1 mg/kg dexamethasone reduces the associated inflammatory reaction and improves prognosis but may cause abortion after day 120. Supportive therapy includes 30 L of warm water containing a rumen stimulant by orogastric tube twice daily.

iv. A 50% recovery rate of early cases is expected.

111 With regard to the Hereford-cross-Friesian heifer in case 110, what control measures would you recommend?

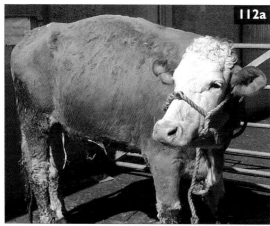

112 A Limousin-cross-Friesian beef cow presents with 5 days' history of inappetance. The cow is dull and depressed and moves slowly around the pen. The cow stands with a roached back with the neck extended and head lowered (112a). The cow has a painful facial expression with the ears back and a fixed glazed stare. On clinical examination the rectal temperature is 39.2°C (102.6°F). The heart rate is 80 beats per minute. No abnormalities are heard during auscultation of the chest. Ruminal movements are depressed, occurring once every 2–3 minutes. The cow appears in discomfort when pressure is applied over the withers but she neither grunts nor dips her back. There are scant dry faeces but no other abnormal findings on rectal examination.

i. What conditions would you consider?
ii. How would you confirm your diagnosis?
iii. What treatment would you administer?
iv. What action would you take?
v. What control measures could be adopted?

111 Control measures include the use of additives for grass silage to produce a more acid pH which discourages multiplication of *L. monocytogenes*. Exclusion of air from the clamp is essential for anaerobic fermentation.

112 i. The most likely conditions to consider include: traumatic reticulitis; localized peritonitis; endocarditis; pleural abscess; liver abscessation; septic pericarditis; chronic suppurative pneumonia; caudal vena cava thrombosis.

ii. Transabdominal ultrasonographic examination immediately caudal to the xiphisternum revealed large quantities of fluid, extending to at least 6 cm, displacing the reticulum from the floor of the abdomen. Numerous large fibrin tags can be observed within this fluid (**112b**).

iii. After 5 days, surgery to remove the wire (if still present within the reticular wall) and treatment of the septic peritonitis with antibiotics will not be successful due to the fibrinous adhesions which markedly reduce reticular contractions and propulsion of digesta.

iv. Euthanasia for welfare reasons is the best option.

v. The prophylactic use of magnets is said to be highly effective in the prevention of traumatic reticulitis in management systems where the disease is common. Outbreaks are described where car tyres with metal rings inlaid in the rubber, used to hold down silage clamp sheeting, have been shredded through forage wagons mixing complete diets. Bonfire sites are another common source of sharp metal objects.

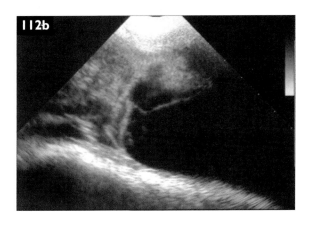

112b

113 A 6-month-old weaned Blackface lamb is brought to the veterinary surgery by a member of the public, having been found near the roadside on open (unfenced) hill ground. The lamb is dull and unable to use its pelvic limbs and adopts a dog-sitting position (113a). There is flaccid paralysis of the pelvic limbs with absent reflexes. There is no tail or rectal tone. Ultrasound examination reveals distension (>8 cm diameter) of the bladder and the rectum is distended with faeces.

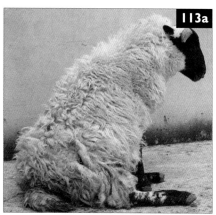

i. What is the extent of the spinal lesion?
ii. What treatments would you administer?
iii. What tests could be undertaken?

114 A five-crop ewe due to lamb in approximately 10 days time presents with a very swollen and oedematous perineum (114). There is no history of this problem in the flock. The ewe is bright and alert with a normal appetite and BCS of 3.0 (scale 1–5). The rectal temperature is normal. The mucous membranes are pink. The udder is very pendulous and there is considerable oedema of the subcutaneous tissue and teats. The perineum is extremely oedematous extending up to 6–8 cm deep giving the overlying skin a translucent appearance.

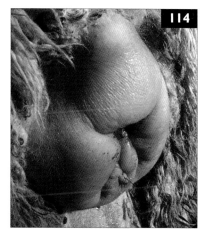

i. What is the probable cause of this condition?
ii. What action would you take?

113 i. Spinal cord compressive lesions (empyema) commonly arise in the vertebral column in the region T2–L3, often at the thoracolumbar (T13/L1) junction causing spastic paralysis and increased spinal reflexes of the pelvic limbs (upper motor neuron signs). Affected sheep adopt a characterisic dog-sitting posture and may attempt to drag themselves using the thoracic limbs. Lesions in the region L4–S2

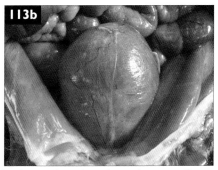

result in flaccid paralysis of the pelvic limbs with reduced or absent reflexes (upper motor neuron signs). Lesions affecting S1–S3 cause hypotonia of the bladder and rectum resulting in distension with urine and faeces, respectively. The lesion extends from L4–S3.

ii. On many hill farms vertebral body abscessation and polyarthritis are not uncommon sequelae to tick-borne fever and tick bite pyaemia. The close proximity to the road and extent of the lesion would be consistent with a traumatic injury. All potential causes of this clinical presentation have a hopeless prognosis.

iii. Radiography could be undertaken to investigate further the cause of the lesion, however the lamb was euthanased immediately because of the guarded prognosis (and cost reasons). Bladder distension was clearly visible at necropsy (113b). Lumbar CSF would be collected from the centre of the lesion.

114 i. The localized nature of the oedema and absence of other clinical signs of congestive heart failure suggest impairment of lymphatic drainage from the perineum. Localized oedema of the vulva can occur after insertion of a Buhner suture to retain a vaginal prolapse but the extent of the oedema is never so pronounced. The shepherd could not recall whether this ewe had had a vaginal prolapse in previous years. The farm has no culling policy for ewes that experience a vaginal prolapse despite recurrence in around 50% of cases.

ii. There is the risk that birth of lambs through the swollen and oedematous posterior reproductive tract could cause tearing of the vaginal mucosa. The ewe was injected intramuscularly with 3 mg dexamethasone. The perineal oedema was greatly reduced 24 hr later. Lambing occurred uneventfully 6 days later with the birth of three live lambs. While there is a slight risk that injection of corticosteroids after day 135 can cause premature birth, the dose rate associated with this is 16 mg (approximately five times that used in this ewe).

115 A 12-day-old Suffolk ram lamb presents 8/10 lame on the right hindlimb. The lameness was noted 3 days ago and the lamb has been injected for 3 consecutive days with amoxicillin/clavulanic acid combination but with little improvement. The right hock joint is hot and painful with an obvious joint effusion. The rectal temperature is 40.2°C (104.4°F). No other joint lesions can

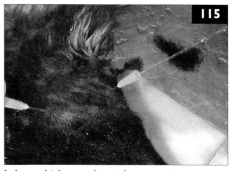

be detected. Arthrocentesis yields a slightly turbid sample with a protein concentration of 21.4 g/L (2.14 g/dL) (normal <3 g/L, < 0.3 g/dL) and a white cell concentration of 26×10^9/L (26×10^3/µL) comprised almost exclusively of neutrophils.

You decide to flush the joint (115).

i. How could effective analgesia be achieved without recourse to general anaesthesia?

ii. What solution would you use to flush the joint, and what volume?

iii. Would you administer antibiotics intra-articularly? If so, which antibiotic?

iv. Would you administer corticosteroids intra-articularly?

v. What follow-up treatment(s) would you recommend?

vi. Is bacteriological culture of the joint fluid valuable in this lamb?

116 A pedigree Texel breeder complains that over the past year or so his prize imported three-shear ram becomes breathless after exertion and now this hyperpnoea sometimes occurs in the ram at rest. The farmer also reports a loss of the ram's body condition over the past few months. Clinical examination reveals exercise intolerance manifested as increased

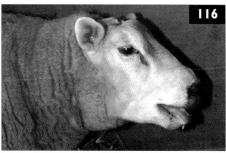

respiratory rate and depth, abdominal expiratory effort, extension of the neck with the head held lowered, and open-mouth breathing (116). There is a slight mucopurulent nasal discharge. On auscultation, although breath sounds are increased in volume, no crackles and wheezes are detected. A dry cough is occasionally noted. The ram is afebrile and no other clinical abnormalities are detected.

i. What conditions would you consider? (Most likely first.)

ii. What tests could be undertaken?

iii. What advice would you offer?

115 i. The lamb is injected with intravenous NSAID. Pelvic limb analgesia is effected by lumbosacral extradural injection of 3 mg/kg of 2% lidocaine solution (1.5 mL for 10 kg lamb).

ii. Hartmann's solution (100–200 mL) is flushed through two 18-gauge needles inserted either side of the patellar ligament into fluid distensions of the joint. The flush is alternated through each needle until the solution runs clear.

iii. Opinion is divided on the use of intra-articular antibiotics. None was used in this case although gentamicin is often used in equine septic joints; crystalline penicillin would be an alternative antibiotic.

iv. Corticosteroids should not be injected intra-articularly in the case of a septic joint.

v. Intramuscular injection of NSAID for 3 consecutive days provides analgesia. Continue amoxicillin/clavulanic acid combination for 10 consecutive days. (Penicillin would be equally effective if the infection is caused by *Streptococcus dysgalactiae*.) The farmer should be instructed to monitor the lamb closely and present it again 3 days after flushing. A second flush may be needed at this time but would indicate a poor prognosis.

vi. Antibiotic therapy prior to culture of the joint fluid may limit the ability to culture the causal organism. Synovial membrane is more likely to yield a positive culture in untreated lambs with joint lesions.

116 i. The most likely conditions to consider include: maedi; laryngeal abscess/pharyngeal abscess; SPA; chronic suppurative pneumonia; CLA causing a mediastinal abscess; lungworm infestation.

ii. The AGID test for MVV proves positive. There are no specific serological tests for the other three main conditions listed; CLA is rare in this clinical presentation. The ram was euthanased and submitted for detailed postmortem examination.

On opening the thoracic cavity the lungs did not collapse. Grossly the lungs were pale, voluminous and weighed 1.6 kg (four times normal weight) in the absence of pulmonary oedema, consolidation or collapse. Small grey spots, 1–2 mm in diameter, were seen subpleurally over all the lung lobes. On sectioning, the lungs had a firm, rubbery texture, the cut surface showed grey spots similar to those seen subpleurally, and was otherwise homogeneous and slightly glassy in appearance. The regional bronchial and caudal mediastinal lymph nodes were 20 times larger than normal with very prominent cortices. Microscopic examination confirmed the diagnosis of maedi.

iii. The farmer should be strongly advised to test all adult stock in his flock for evidence of maedi-visna infection using the AGID test. In this case, 30% of all adult sheep were seropositive. The farmer was strongly advised to cull all seropositive sheep and their offspring and initiate a regular test and slaughter policy.

117 An 8-month-old pedigree Suffolk ram lamb presents with 1 month's history of unilateral scrotal swelling and stiff gait. There is loss of wool on the affected side of the scrotum (117a). No other abnormalities are noted on clinical examination.

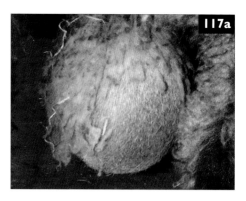

i. What conditions would you consider?
ii. What further tests could be undertaken?
iii. What control measures could be introduced on this stud farm?

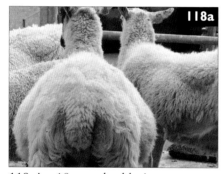

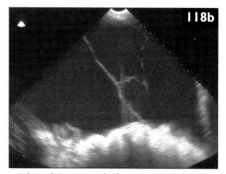

118 An 18-month-old gimmer presents with a history of chronic weight loss (BCS 1.5) while the remainder of sheep in the group are within a range of 3–3.5. The rectal temperature is 39.0°C (102.2°F). The sheep has a reduced appetite. There is no diarrhoea. At rest the ewe is tachypnoeic (40 breaths per minute). Auscultation of the chest reveals no abnormalities except a slight increase in heart rate (96 beats per minute). There is considerable abdominal enlargement (118a) with an obvious fluid thrill. There is effusion affecting both hock joints.

Ultrasonographic examination (5.0 MHz sector transducer connected to a real-time, B-mode ultrasound machine) reveals dorsal displacement of abdominal viscera by 10–12 cm of fluid, hepatomegaly with changes consistent with chronic venous congestion, and slight fibrin tags on the liver capsule (118b).

i. What conditions would you consider?
ii. What further tests would you undertake?
iii. What is your diagnosis and what treatment would you administer?

117 i. The most likely conditions to consider include: epididymitis; scrotal hernia; orchitis; haematoma. Palpation reveals normal spermatic cords and neck of the scrotum. No hernia is identified. The left testicle is slightly smaller than normal but is freely moveable within the scrotal sac. The right

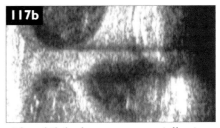

testicle/epididymis is swollen and hard with a bilobed appearance. Adhesions prevent free movement of the right testicle and a discharging sinus is present on the ventral pole. Clinical findings are consistent with right-sided epididymitis.

ii. Further tests could include: ultrasonography; cytology and bacteriology of ejaculate. Examination using a 5 MHz linear scanner reveals a grossly enlarged head of the right epididymis with numerous 1–3 cm diameter anechoic areas consistent with abscesses (117b). *Histophilus seminis* is the most common cause of such lesions in the UK. In countries with endemic *Brucella ovis* infection detection of large numbers of white cells in the ejaculate, in addition to a high percentage of detached sperm heads (>20%) may be the first indication of infection.

iii. The diagnosis is epididymitis possibly caused by *Histophilus seminis*. This ram lamb should be culled; unilateral castration is ill advised. Male sheep should be maintained in small groups in a clean environment, fencing off dirty areas where rams typically congregate. Irrigation of the prepuce with diluted antiseptic solutions as lambs reach puberty may limit bacterial colonization. Oral chlortetracycline given in feed daily for several months around puberty is widely used for *B. ovis* control, parenteral oxytetracycline could be used similarly.

118 i. Possible conditions include: right-sided heart failure as a consequence of bacterial endocarditis involving the tricuspid valve or increased resistance in the lung field; subacute fluke infestation but only one sheep affected; adenocarcinoma of the small intestine with transcoelomic spread impairing lymphatic drainiage; chronic peritonitis; ascites as a consequence of low serum albumin concentration.

ii. Further tests include routine haematology, serum protein analysis, and peritoneal fluid analysis. In this case, routine haematology reveals normal values. Serum protein analysis reveals marginally low albumin but normal globulin concentrations. Peritoneal fluid analysis reveals a modified transudate (protein concentration 34.8 g/L, 3.48 g/dL) with a normal white cell count with few neutrophils.

iii. The most likely diagnosis is bacterial endocarditis although this cannot be conclusively proven. Treatment for 6 weeks with daily procaine penicillin can be attempted, but the prognosis is grave. Euthanasia for welfare reasons is indicated.

119 An 18-month-old homebred ram presents with a large firm subcutaneous swelling below the angle of the right mandible (119a) which has been noted by the farmer for the past 2 weeks. The swelling has not reduced in size despite 4 consecutive days' treatment with procaine penicillin. Inspection reveals no skin lesions in other rams in the group.
i. What is your diagnosis? (Most likely first.)
ii. What would you do?

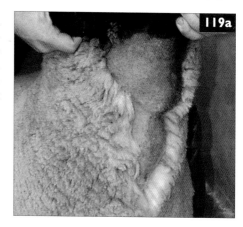

120 In mid-winter a sheep farmer client receives a report of 'pneumonia' (120) in a batch of 9-month-old lambs sent to a local slaughter plant. When questioned further the farmer reports a lot of coughing in the remaining lambs left to market. The lambs were housed 8 weeks ago and are fed *ad libitum* concentrates. The lambs were vaccinated against clostridial disease at 4 and 5 months old but not pasteurella pneumonia.

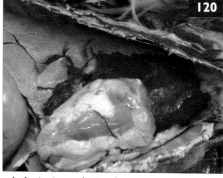

The lambs were last treated with an anthelmintic early in the previous autumn, 1 month before housing. A large amount of coughing is present whenever the lambs are disturbed but they appear bright and alert. Examination of three lambs with an elevated respiratory rate (60 breaths per minute) reveals a normal rectal temperature (39.2–39.6°C (102.6–103.3°F)). The ocular mucous membranes are congested with episcleral injection in one of the three lambs but this is attributable to IKC which affects about 10% of lambs in the group. None of the lambs has a mucopurulent nasal discharge.
i. What conditions would you suspect?
ii. What treatments would you administer?
iii. What advice would you give?

119 i. The most likely conditions to consider include: deep-seated abscess; cellulitis; actinobacillosis; phlebitis/perivascular injection; CLA affecting the submandibular lymph node.
ii. Ultrasound examination using a 5 MHz linear scanner reveals a 4 cm capsule surrounding a large 8 cm diameter abscess (**119b**). A viscous green discharge is obtained after aspiration with a 5 cm 14-gauge needle. The centre

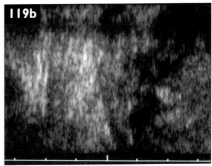

of the lesion is lanced with a 22 scalpel blade, irrigated with dilute antiseptic solution, and a gauze swab is inserted into the incision to prevent it sealing over. The abscess is irrigated daily for 3 more days, inserting a new gauze plug each day to prevent the incision healing over. The lesion resolved and no further treatment was necessary. Bacteriological examination of a dry cotton swab taken from the abscess before irrigation yielded *Arcanobacterium pyogenes* and not *Corynebacterium pseudotuberculosis* (the causal organism of CLA). In the UK, CLA most commonly affects the parotid lymph nodes. In other countries CLA produces lung and liver lesions. Fighting injuries to the poll regions and drainage parotid lymph node lesions are unique to the UK.

120 i. The most likely conditions to consider would include: atypical pneumonia (Mycoplasma-type; cuffing pneumonia); *Mannheimia haemolytica* associated with viral type pneumonia (possibly parainfluenza 3 virus); lungworm.
ii. The farmer was advised to inject any inappetant lambs with a single injection of long-acting oxytetracycline intramuscularly, strictly observing meat withholding times. An increased respiratory rate and occasional coughing were not considered sufficient criteria to warrant immediate antibiotic therapy. Faeces from the three lambs failed to reveal any lungworm larvae (Baermann technique). The mild clinical signs and low morbidity rate indicated that there was no requirement for metaphylactic antibiotic injection.
iii. Improved ventilation and reduced stocking may reduce the extent of enzootic pneumonia but this disease does not usually impact upon health and production. Vaccination against pasteurellosis would be most effective if completed before weaning when most losses caused by *Pasteurella trehalosi* occur. A live attenuated intranasal bovine parainfluenza 3 vaccine given to 1–2-week-old lambs is reported to be highly effective in reducing respiratory disease, particularly in those flocks where lambs are housed for the first few months of life, but may not be effective in this disease situation.

121 A farmer complains of apparent sudden-onset profound depression and blindness in 12 of 300 6-month-old lambs. When confined, the lambs are found head-pressing (121a) and there is frequent teeth-grinding. There are no cranial nerve deficits. The lambs are poorly grown (18–24 kg) with a dirty open fleece. The lambs have poor abdominal fill and there is faecal staining of

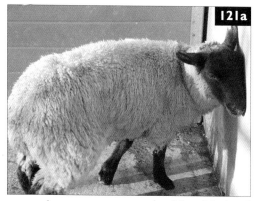

the perineum and tail. The lambs are grazing permanent grassland in a National Park used extensively by the general public for walking their dogs.

i. What conditions would you consider?
ii. How would you investigate this problem?
iii. What treatments would you administer?
iv. How would you prevent a similar problem next year?

122 A yearling female sheep (hogg) presents at your surgery with a cervicovaginal prolapse during first-stage labour. The hogg is straining vigorously and in considerable distress. The vaginal mucosa is congested, oedematous, friable, and dirty (122). Fetal membranes protrude through the cervix which is dilated to approximately 2 cm.

i. How will you effect proper analgesia in this case?
ii. What action will you take?
iii. What are the economics of your proposed action plan?

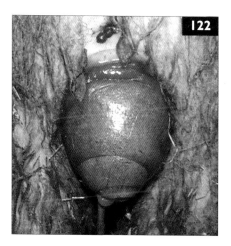

121 i. The most likely conditions to consider include: severe cobalt deficiency causing white liver disease; PEM; sulphur toxicity; subacute fasciolosis; sarcocystosis; hepatotoxin; acute coenurosis; focal symmetrical encephalomalacia. The poor growth rates of this group of lambs could be the result of poor grazing, overstocking, PGE, and trace element

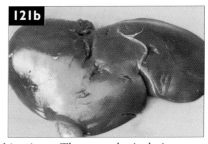

deficiency acting alone or in various combinations. The neurological signs are consistent with a diffuse cortical lesion – most likely a hepatic encephalopathy.

ii. Faecal worm egg counts average 400 epg. No fluke eggs are seen. Liver enzyme concentrations (AST, GLDH, and GGT) are raised four- to six-fold in the four lambs sampled. Serum vitamin B_{12} concentration from six lambs reveal very low levels (mean <88.6 pmol/L, <120 pg/mL).

iii. All lambs should be treated with vitamin B_{12} by intramuscular injection. The worst affected lambs were given 4 L of diluted oral rehydration solution by orogastric tube to stimulate appetite. Two of 12 lambs failed to respond to vitamin B_{12} and supportive therapy and were euthanased for welfare reasons. Necropsy revealed a pale and friable liver (**121b**).

iv. The low unit cost of cobalt sulphate allows routine inclusion in anthelmintic drenches (commercial 'SC' preparations, or at inclusion rates of 15–30 g per 10 L of 2.25% benzimidazole or 1.5% levamisole drench).

122 i. Flunixin meglumine (or another NSAID) is injected intravenously. The hogg is injected with a combination of lidocaine plus xylazine at the sacrococcygeal site to allow replacement of the oedematous cervicovaginal prolapse and insertion of the Buhner retention suture. The first intercoccygeal space is identified by digital palpation during slight vertical movement of the tail, and a 25 mm 19-gauge needle is directed at 20° to the tail which is held horizontally. Correct position of the needle is determined by the lack of resistance to injection of 2% lidocaine (0.5–0.6 mg/kg injected over 10 s; 1.25 mL for a 50 kg hogg) and 0.07 mg/kg xylazine (0.2 mL for a 50 kg hogg). The hogg is also injected with 44,000 IU/kg of procaine penicillin prior to surgery.

ii. Perform a caesarean operation. Any attempt to dilate the cervix using digital pressure over 10–20 minutes will almost certainly cause rupture of the friable vaginal mucosa/cervix. Effective flank analgesia is achieved following distal paravertebral block using 2% lidocaine.

iii. Cost of the caesarean operation is approximately one third of the market value for a hogg with a single lamb.

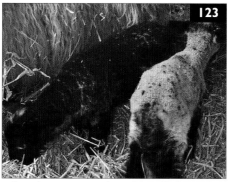

123 You are presented with a gaunt 8-day-old Suffolk-cross castrated male lamb. The lamb has been noted to be very dull and inappetant for the past 2 days. The lamb is in much poorer condition, smaller, and less active than its co-twin (123). The rectal temperature is marginally subnormal (38.2°C (100.8°F)). The heart rate is 90 beats per minute. The mucous membranes appear congested. The respiratory rate is increased to 40 breaths per minute. The umbilicus remains wet. Abdominal palpation reveals gas-filled abomasum and loops of small intestine. The ewe shows no evidence of mastitis to account for the lamb's poor condition.
i. What conditions would you consider in your differential diagnosis list?
ii. What further examination could be undertaken?
iii. What treatment would you administer?
iv. How could this condition be prevented?

Perinatal lamb mortality (%) in relation to litter size (singles, twins, and triplets) and dam nutritional plane (low, medium, and high) during late gestation			
	Low	Medium	High
Singles	0	7.1	0
Twins	18.0	13.8	0
Triplets	41.6	27.0	22.2

124 Research work undertaken in commercial flocks almost 40 years ago established the direct link between litter size and nutritional plane of the ewe during late gestation with perinatal lamb mortality.

How can you use these data to advise your sheep clients regarding husbandry and feeding practices today?

123 i. The most likely conditions to consider include: peritonitis following umbilical infection; hepatic necrobacillosis; infected urachus; starvation; wool balls (trichobezoars).

ii. In hepatic necrobacillosis the umbilical vessels may be palpable (greater than pencil diameter) extending craniodorsally; the liver lobes may be palpable behind the costal arch but these features are not always present. Ultrasound examination may detect focal lesions within the liver parenchyma suggestive of abscessation. Localized accumulations of inflammatory exudate may be imaged in the case of peritonitis but often reaction is restricted to fibrinous adhesions.

iii. The lamb should be euthanased for welfare reasons and the cause of illness determined at necropsy.

iv. Postmortem examination revealed numerous liver abscesses and associated localized peritonitis with fibrinous adhesions between gas-distended loops of small intestine. The umbilicus must be immersed in strong iodine solution within 15 minutes after birth, and again 4–6 hr later.

124 As the average UK weaning percentage for lowground flocks is only 155%, a scanning percentage of 205% between days 45–90 of pregnancy with 20–25% of the flock with triplets makes little sense. Why flush ewes before mating to achieve higher ovulation, implantation and lambing rates when triplet lambs have a much higher mortality rate? Triplet-bearing ewes are much more prone to pregnancy toxaemia, ruptured prepubic tendon, and vaginal prolapse. Perhaps a less prolific breed/hybrid should be selected.

Ewes should be grouped on litter size and fed accordingly. Serum 3-OH butyrate concentrations of twin- and triplet-bearing ewes should be determined 5–6 weeks before lambing to quantify energy status and diet corrected accordingly. The energy status is reassessed 2 weeks later to monitor the situation. The extra 2–4 MJ/head/day necessary to correct the diet from low to high nutritional plane for the last 6 weeks of gestation in many flocks costs very little per head yet could halve perinatal losses. The advisory work developed by Dr Angus Russel 40 years ago is greatly underutilized by veterinary practitioners today. Such advice is the cornerstone of all sheep health plans and can make a major contribution to sheep health and welfare.

The weakest triplet lambs must be removed soon after birth (after ingesting colostrum) and reared artificially from a few hours old. Cross-fostered triplet lambs may struggle to keep up with a vigorous singleton even if adoption is successful. When 'lamb adopters' become necessary for 5–7 days, all that may be achieved is a severe check to the ewe's milk production and her own lamb's growth rate.

125 Halfway through lambing time a sheep client complains of high morbidity and mortality in 24–36-hr-old lambs showing excess salivation with a wet lower jaw, cold mouth and poor suck reflex, and retained meconium (125a). There is progressive abdominal distension with fluid and gas. The rectal temperature is subnormal. There is dehydration, poor peripheral perfusion with cold extremities, and a rapid weak pulse during the agonal stages.

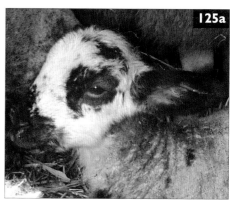

i. What conditions would you consider?
ii. What treatments would you recommend?
iii. What control measures would you instigate?

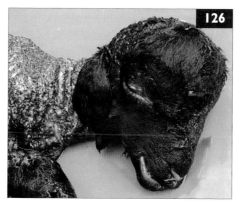

126 A farmer reports seven malformed lambs (126) from 60 pedigree Suffolk ewes. Affected lambs have marked doming of the skull (hypertensive hydrocephalus) that has caused dystocia. Affected lambs are either stillborn or die within hours. The cases have included twins in which either both lambs are affected or only one lamb; the unaffected twin lamb has grown and behaved normally. This problem has never occurred before in this flock.

i. What is your diagnosis?
ii. What advice would you offer?

125 i. The most likely conditions to consider include: endotoxaemia (watery mouth disease); septicaemia; *Escherichia coli* enteritis (enterotoxigenic strains); starvation/mismothering/exposure (SME complex); cryptosporidiosis.

Clinical chemistry reveals low plasma glucose concentration and leucopenia, but elevated lactate and BUN concentrations consistent with endotoxaemia.

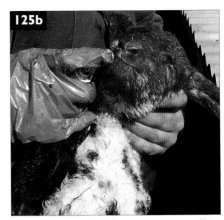

ii. Despite abomasal distension, oral rehydration solution administration (50 mL/kg four times daily) by stomach tube is essential. Many lambs showing disease are bacteraemic therefore a broad-spectrum antibiotic (amoxicillin, oxytetracycline) should be injected intramuscularly. Flunixin meglumine should be given intravenously to counter the endotoxaemia.

iii. Control measures include improving hygiene standards in the lambing shed and ensuring passive antibody transfer. Paraformaldehyde powder should be applied daily to the straw bedding. Individual pens should have a concrete base and must be cleaned out completely, disinfected, and allowed to dry between ewes. The most effective means of preventing watery mouth disease is giving an oral antibiotic preparation (an aminoglycoside such as spectinomycin) within 15 minutes of birth (125b). In the early stages of watery mouth disease, soapy water enemas and mild laxatives/purgatives are often effective. Metaclopramide is too expensive.

126 i. The most likely diagnosis is Dandy–Walker malformation (agenesis of the caudal cerebellar vermis). There is marked distension of the ventricular system including the lateral ventricles, the third and fourth ventricles. Hydrocephalus with agenesis of the cerebellar vermis is consistent features of the Dandy–Walker malformation. The prevalence of Dandy–Walker malformation can be high with 16 affected lambs from 22 ewes in one report.

ii. An investigation of Dandy–Walker malformation in three flocks revealed the condition only occurred in Suffolk sheep and was associated with particular rams, although exposure to an unidentified teratogen could not be excluded. Careful examination of breeding records in this pedigree flock identified all affected lambs as the progeny of a ram introduced into the flock for that breeding season. It would be prudent that this ram, and his progeny, were not used for further breeding purposes.

127 In late summer a farmer complains that some ewes have lost considerable condition as a consequence of not grazing and are observed frequently kicking at their heads with their hindfeet, causing serious damage to the poll and ears (127; compare to the other sheep in the photograph). The affected ewes seem distressed, frequently running 10–15 m then stopping, only to start running away again.

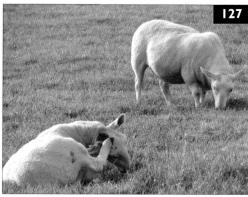

i. What are possible causes of this problem? (Most likely cause first.)
ii. How can this problem be controlled?

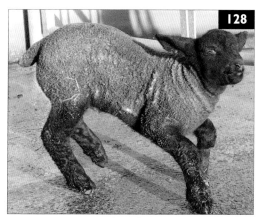

128 In early spring you are presented with two 1-month-old Suffolk lambs with tetraparesis of 10 days' duration. The rectal temperature of each lamb is normal. There are no joint swellings and no swollen lymph nodes. The lambs appear to show signs of cervical pain with 'the head tucked into their shoulders' but gentle manipulation is not resented (128). The reflex arcs are normal in all four limbs.
i. What is your diagnosis? (Most likely first.)
ii. What treatments would you administer?
iii. How could you confirm your diagnosis?
iv. What preventive measures could be adopted?

127 i. Feeding around head wounds and ear tag injuries (and horn base) by the muscid fly *Hydrotea irritans* causes considerable irritation that frequently results in self-trauma. Grazing patterns are disturbed and affected sheep often isolate themselves and remain in shade where available. They may stand with the head held lowered with frequent head shaking and ear movements. Alternatively, sheep adopt a submissive posture in sternal recumbency with the neck extended and the head held on the ground. Kicking at the head often greatly exacerbates damage caused by headflies to the horn base, and such action may also traumatize the skin of the neck and ears (**127**). Head rubbing also causes considerable self-trauma. Bleeding and serum exudation attract more flies and aggravate the problem. There is rapid loss of condition in severely affected sheep. Myiasis may result in some cases.

ii. Housing is essential for sheep with large skin lesions to allow time for complete healing. Topical emollients and antibiotic preparations are not usually necessary and skin wounds heal well provided flies are denied access to these areas. Pour-on fly control preparations, such as high cis cypermethrin or deltamethrin, must be applied before the anticipated headfly season and especially to horned sheep. Such treatments should be repeated every 3–4 weeks during the fly season or as directed by the data sheet instructions.

128 i. The most likely conditions to consider include: vertebral empyema C1–C6; *Streptococcus dysgalactiae* infection of the atlanto-occipital joint causing cord compression, although these are older than usual cases; muscular dystrophy (white muscle disease); delayed swayback. In the delayed form of swayback (enzootic ataxia) the lambs are normal at birth but show progressive weakness of the pelvic limbs from 2–4 months of age. Signs are often first noted during gathering or movement when affected lambs lag behind the remainder of the flock. The pelvic limbs are weak with reduced muscle tone and reflexes, and show muscle atrophy. Lumbar CSF protein concentration is normal in this lamb, ruling out significant cord compression from an inflammatory focus.

ii. There is limited evidence that copper supplementation of lambs with enzootic ataxia slows progress of the condition. Both lambs were treated with copper; one of which recovered fully.

iii. Although a very unusual clinical presentation, delayed swayback was confirmed by histopathological examination of the spinal cord in the lamb euthanased for welfare reasons.

iv. Prevention of swayback by copper supplementation of ewes during mid-pregnancy must very carefully consider the prevalence of confirmed or suspected swayback cases in the flock (two of 150 lambs), breed of sheep (Suffolk – susceptible to copper toxicity), supplementary feeding during gestation (winter 2006 unique as extremely mild), and geographical area, including soil analysis.

129 A 4-year-old Rouge de L'Ouest ram presents with 3 months' history of 'collapse' when stressed such as gathering by a sheepdog. The ram assumes sternal recumbency with the neck extended and the head held on the ground (129) for up to 10 minutes' duration. In this state the sheep cannot be prompted to regain its feet but will do so unaided soon afterwards and appear normal. Postural and gait abnormalities include pelvic limb ataxia but with preservation of muscle strength, dysmetria, most commonly hypermetria of the thoracic limbs, and a wide-based stance. The gait abnormalities are most obvious when the animal is made to trot downhill or turn acute angles, when hopping with both pelvic limbs is frequently observed.

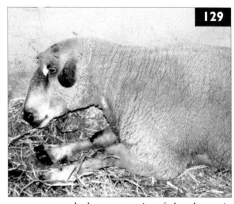

i. What conditions would you consider? (Most likely first.)
ii. How could you establish a definitive diagnosis?
iii. What treatment(s) would you administer?
iv. What control measures would you recommend?

130 A two-crop ewe from a group of 155 pastured sheep due to start lambing in 3 weeks has aborted two fresh fetuses. Three other abortions have occurred over the previous 5 days. The ewe is bright and alert but there is a red–brown vulval discharge over the wool of the tail and perineum (130). The rectal temperature is 40.0°C (104.0°F). The udder is reasonably well developed and there is some accumulated colostrum.

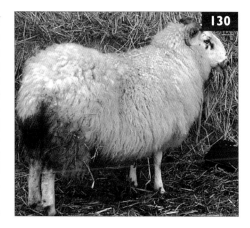

i. What samples would you collect?
ii. List the common causes of abortion.
iii. What treatments would you consider?
iv. What control measures could be adopted?

129 i. The most likely conditions to consider include: scrapie; cervical vertebral malformation; cerebellar abiotrophy.
ii. There are confirmatory antemortem tests for scrapie but they are not used for clinical diagnosis at present. The clinical diagnosis is confirmed by histopathological examination of brain tissue at necropsy with the demonstration of characteristic neuronal vacuolation and astrocytic hypertrophy. The collection of a normal CSF sample from suspected scrapie cases may assist in eliminating those bacterial and viral infections of the CNS that evoke an intrathecal inflammatory reaction.
iii. There is no treatment for scrapie and affected sheep should be euthanased as soon as the condition is suspected on clinical examination.
iv. Regulatory authorities should be informed of suspected scrapie cases as appropriate. Following confirmation of scrapie in a flock, control is based upon genetic selection for resistance by determining three common polymorphisms. Genotyping services are available worldwide.

130 i. A vaginal swab, fetuses, and placentae should be submitted for laboratory examination. Blood samples are collected from all aborted ewes for toxoplasma and EAE serology.
ii. Common abortifacient agents include: *Chlamydophila psittaci* (EAE); salmonellosis including *Salmonella montevideo*, *S. typhimurium*, and other serotypes; *Campylobacter fetus fetus*; *Toxoplasma gondii*; *Listeria monocytogenes*; *Pasteurella* spp.; tick-borne fever.
   C. psittaci was demonstrated in direct smears from the placentae and a strong positive titre obtained in three of four blood samples; a very high titre for toxoplasma was recorded for the other ewe. Any further aborted material must be submitted to monitor the situation. The zoonotic risk of chlamydial abortion, especially to pregnant women, should be stressed.
iii. The ewe was treated with intravenous oxytetracycline and made a rapid recovery. The ewe accepted a small male triplet foster lamb. All ewes in the group were injected with 20 mg/kg long-acting oxytetracycline intramuscularly that same day to reduce further abortions.
iv. Aborted ewes must be isolated for at least 6 weeks and all aborted material buried or burned. With EAE now present in the flock the farmer should be strongly advised to vaccinate all replacement females even if purchasing EAE-accredited stock. In this case it was recommended that all ewes which had possibly encountered infection this spring should also be vaccinated, and treated with long-acting oxytetracycline next year 6 weeks and 3 weeks before lambing. Vaccination against toxoplasmosis would depend upon titres in aborted versus control ewes.

131 A 4-month-old Suffolk-cross lamb is found recumbent, dull, and depressed (131), and separated from its dam. The rectal temperature is 41.1°C (106.6°F). The respiratory rate is 24 breaths per minute and the heart rate is 120 beats per minute. There are no ocular or nasal discharges. The mucous membranes appear congested. Auscultation of the chest reveals increased

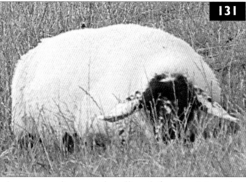

wheezes anteroventrally. The lamb has passed normal pelleted faeces. No other clinical abnormalities are detected.

i. What conditions would you consider? (Most likely first.)
ii. What treatment would you recommend?
iii. What control measures could be adopted?

132 A Texel ewe presents with 2 days' history of lateral recumbency and inability to raise itself even when assisted (132). When supported the ewe has a normal appetite but is unable to maintain sternal recumbency. The ewe is bright and alert with no cranial nerve deficits. The head is held in the normal position and there is no evidence of pain associated with gentle manipulation of the cervical vertebrae or increased muscular tone in the neck region. The

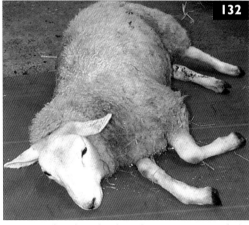

local reflex arcs involving the thoracic and pelvic limbs (determination of the withdrawal and tendon reflexes) are increased, suggestive of a lesion C2–C6.

i. What conditions would you consider? (Most likely first.)
ii. What tests would you undertake to confirm your suspicions?

131 i. The most likely conditions to consider include: acute respiratory disease (*Mannheimia haemolytica*); septicaemia; early stage of clostridial disease, e.g. pulpy kidney disease; nephrosis.

ii. The lamb is treated with 20 mg/kg oxytetracycline injected intravenously. The lamb was considerably improved by the following morning and was treated for 2 more days with 10 mg/kg oxytetracycline injected intramuscularly. Tilmicosin could have been used as an alternative antibiotic.

iii. Vaccination of the dam with a pasteurella vaccine will provide some passively derived immunity for the first 4 weeks or so of life. Thereafter, vaccination of lambs from 3 weeks old is required to provide active immunity. Two vaccinations are required 4–6 weeks apart. Thus, despite undertaking a vaccination programme, lambs may remain susceptible to pasteurellosis in that period between the waning of passively derived immunity and active immunity following two vaccinations.

Although not licensed for use in sheep in all countries, lambs can be vaccinated with a live attenuated bovine parainfluenza 3 intranasal vaccine once only from about 2 weeks old.

132 i. The most likely conditions to consider include: trauma or fracture of one or more cervical vertebrae; cervical vertebral empyema; aberrant injection in neck region tracking to affect cervical spinal cord; cervical vertebral malformation; sarcocystosis.

ii. CSF analysis could be carried out. Inspection of lumbosacral CSF collected under local anaesthesia revealed no pathological haemorrhage or xanthochromic change. Laboratory analysis revealed a markedly elevated protein concentration of 2.4 g/L (0.24 g/dL) (normal <0.3 g/L, <0.03 g/dL) and an increased white cell concentration comprising mainly of lymphocytes. A provisional diagnosis of a compressive cervical spinal lesion of nontraumatic aetiology was made, possibly vertebral empyema, and the ewe was destroyed for humane reasons.

Pathological lesions were confined to the cervical spinal cord where a white, firm elliptically shaped mass (measuring approximately 1 × 3 cm) was present subdurally overlying the spinal cord on the right side extending over spinal segments C2 and C3. The spinal cord tissue was compressed but not invaded and the overlying dura mater was intact. Histological examination revealed the lesion had the appearance of a rapidly growing fibroma or fibrosarcoma derived from meninges. The mitotic rate of the tumour was extremely high (28 mitotic figures per 10 high power fields) and this, together with the areas of necrosis, indicated that the tumour was growing rapidly.

133 You are presented with a recumbent Scottish Blackface lamb (133a). The previous day the farmer noted that the lamb was blind and wandered aimlessly. There was marked dorsiflexion of the neck ('star-gazing'). The sheep is hyperaesthetic to auditory and tactile stimuli which precipitate seizure activity. Dorsomedial strabismus and spontaneous horizontal nystagmus are present. There is no menace

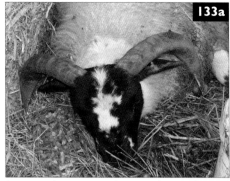

response in either eye. No other abnormalities are detected on clinical examination.

i. What conditions would you consider?
ii. What treatment would you administer?
iii. What is the prognosis for this case?
iv. How can the diagnosis be confirmed?
v. What control measures would you recommend?

134 In mid-spring your client complains of weight loss and diarrhoea affecting at least 30 of 120 3–6-week-old Suffolk-cross lambs (134); the ewes are unaffected. The lambs were reared indoors for the first few weeks of life then turned out approximately 2 weeks ago to permanent pasture. The ewes are fed 1 kg of 18% crude protein concentrate per head per day plus access to clamp silage in a

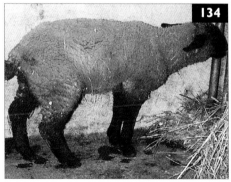

feed bunk. The younger lambs are more severely affected and appear in poor bodily condition with considerable faecal staining of the tail and perineum. There is frequent tenesmus with the passage of small quantities of fluid faeces containing a large amount of mucus and flecks of fresh blood.

i. What common problems would you consider? (Most likely first.)
ii. How could you confirm your provisional diagnosis?
iii. What treatment would you administer?

133 i. The most likely conditions to consider would include: PEM (synonym cerebrocortical necrosis); focal symmetrical encephalomalacia; meningitis/brain abscess; listerial meningoencephalitis.

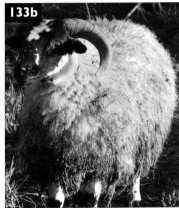

ii. Treatment for PEM includes the intravenous injection of thiamine (10 mg/kg twice daily) on the first occasion, then by the intramuscular route twice daily for 2 more days. There is evidence from field studies that intravenous injection of 1.0 mg/kg of dexamethasone, or similar short-acting corticosteroid, aids recovery by reducing brain swelling.

iii. The prognosis is good when sheep are presented early in the clinical course; this sheep made a rapid recovery (133b).

iv. Diagnosis is based upon the rapid response to timely thiamine treatment. Diagnostic biochemical parameters for PEM, including thiaminase activities in blood, rumen fluid or faeces, are rarely used in farm animal practice. At necrospy affected areas of the cortex may exhibit a bright white autofluoresence when cut sections are viewed under ultraviolet light (Wood's lamp; 365 nm). This property has been attributed to the accumulation of lipofuchsin in macrophages but not all PEM cases fluoresce. Definitive diagnosis relies upon the histological findings in the cortical lesions of vacuolation and cavitation of the ground substance with astrocytic swelling, neuronal shrinkage, and necrosis.

v. Disease occurs sporadically and there are no specific control measures. Prompt recognition and treatment are vital.

134 i. The most likely conditions to consider include: coccidiosis; cryptosporidiosis; *Strongyloides papillosus* infestation; salmonellosis; nematodiriasis.

ii. The clinical signs are suggestive of coccidiosis. Oocyst counts can be variable but are usually very high in lambs scouring for more than several days. Identification of the pathogenic species *Eimeria ovinoidalis* or *E. crandallis* is rarely undertaken. Gut smears and histopathology of gut sections are taken from dead lambs. The response to treatment for coccidiosis helps to confirm the diagnosis.

iii. Treatment options include a single drench with diclazuril or decoquinate added to the lambs' concentrate ration, which can be used as a treatment/preventive measure. Where doubts exist over feed intake, diclazuril is the treatment of choice. The feeding areas and water trough area can become very heavily contaminated, therefore the sheep should be moved to a clean field immediately.

135 In late summer a pedigree Suffolk shearling ram presents in severe respiratory distress with its head lowered and the neck extended (135a). The ram's respiratory rate is increased to 90 breaths per minute with a marked inspiratory noise (honking) audible 10 yards away from the animal. The nostrils are flared and the mouth is held open with the tongue partially protruded and frothy saliva around the mouth and lower jaw. The rectal temperature is 40.2°C (104.4°F). The mucous membranes appear cyanotic. Auscultation over the larynx reveals very loud crackles transferred over the

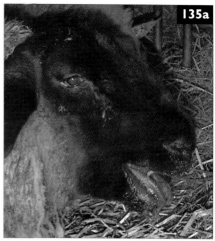

whole lung field. The heart rate is increased to 120 beats per minute.
i. What conditions would you consider? (Most likely first.)
ii. How could you confirm your diagnosis?
iii. What actions/treatments would you recommend?
iv. What control measures would you recommend?

136 A 2-week-old lamb is very dull and weak, and in much worse bodily condition than its twin. The lamb stands with its head held lowered and has a roached back stance (136). The rectal temperature is subnormal (38.0°C (100.4°F)). The heart rate is 90 beats per minute. The mucous membranes are congested. The respiratory rate is increased to 40 breaths per minute. No abnormal sounds are heard on auscultation of

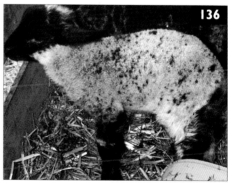

the chest. Careful abdominal palpation over the umbilicus and caudal to the xiphisternum elicits a painful response. There is no evidence of diarrhoea.
i. What conditions would you consider?
ii. What treatment would you administer?
iii. What control measures could be adopted?

135 i. The most likely conditions to consider include: laryngeal chondritis; laryngeal foreign body; enlarged retropharyngeal lymph nodes/ pharyngeal abscess; pasteurellosis.

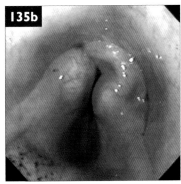

ii. Swelling of the arytenoids, with or without erosion/infection of the overlying epithelium, causing severe narrowing of the larynx can be visualized on endoscopic examination (135b) but this procedure should not be undertaken in severely dyspnoeic sheep.

iii. Treatment includes 10 mg dexamethasone injected intravenously immediately to reduce laryngeal oedema. There are few data to indicate which antibiotic is most appropriate; *Arcanobacterium pyogenes* is commonly isolated from lesions. Early recognition and a prolonged primary course of antibiotics are essential; the recovery rate of relapsed cases is low. In emergency situations an emergency tracheostomy can be performed under local anaesthesia via a ventral midline approach in the mid-cervical region. It may prove difficult fixing the trachea to make the incision between two tracheal rings. Intranasal/transtracheal oxygen administration via a wide bore needle can be supplied if available. Be aware that abscessation of the arytenoid cartilage(s) may be present and that no treatment will successfully resolve this problem.

iv. Laryngeal chondritis is common in Beltex, Texel, and Suffolk rams. Conformation and turbulent air passage through the oedematous larynx of rams approaching the breeding season leads to erosion of the lining epithelium, with secondary bacterial infection causing swelling and further narrowing of the airway. The level of concentrate feeding should be reduced when preparing rams for sale. These potential causes are challenged when the condition occurs in ewes! There may be a heritable component.

136 i. The most likely conditions to consider include: hepatic necrobacillosis; localized peritonitis associated with umbilical infection; suppurative pneumonia.

ii. Treatment of the *Fusobacterium necrophorum* infection with antibiotics (procaine penicillin) could be attempted but the prognosis for this lamb is hopeless and it should be euthanased for welfare reasons.

iii. Control measures include immersion of the lamb's navel in strong veterinary iodine BP within the first 15 minutes of birth and 2–4 hr later to prevent ascending infection of the umbilical remnant. In housed sheep, regular addition of clean straw bedding is essential throughout the lambing period. Paraformaldehyde powder sprinkled on the bedding helps to limit contamination of the lambing environment.

137 A ram presents with 5 days' history of ataxia and hyperaesthesia to tactile stimuli. The ram is inappetant with an elevated rectal temperature (40.5°C (104.9°F)), and spends long periods in sternal recumbency with the neck extended and the head held lowered. The menace response and pupillary light reflexes are normal. There are no detectable cranial nerve deficits. The ram displays a wide-based stance (137). There is marked hypermetria involving all four limbs and ataxia of the pelvic limbs but there is preserva-

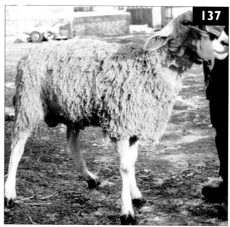

tion of limb muscle strength. Spinal reflexes of the thoracic and pelvic limbs are normal.

i. What area(s) of the central nervous system is involved in the disease process?
ii. How could this be further investigated?
iii. What treatments would you administer?
iv. What is the prognosis?

138 In early summer you are presented at the surgery with an 8-week-old pet Texel-cross ram lamb with a rectal prolapse. The lamb has been reared with three other lambs in a garden and fed *ad libitum* concentrates. The rectal prolapse extends for approximately 8 cm and is markedly oedematous but not traumatized (138). The mucous membranes appear normal and the lamb is not dehydrated. The respiratory rate is 22 breaths per minute and the heart rate is 90 beats per minute. The abdomen appears slightly distended. No rumen sounds are heard over 2 minutes.

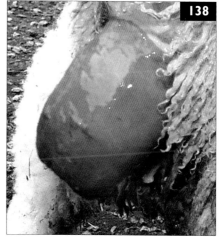

i. How will you deal with this problem?
ii. What conditions may have predisposed to rectal prolapse in this lamb? (Most likely first.)

137 i. The cerebellum is the likely site of the disease process. Conditions which could cause the clinical signs include: cerebellar abscess/focal meningitis; cerebellar abiotrophy; gid cyst involving the cerebellum; sarcocystosis involving the cerebellum. A cervical spinal lesion is another possible diagnosis (e.g. fracture C2–C6); cervical spinal lesions would present with weakness affecting all four limbs, and possibly pain when manipulating the sheep's head/neck. Scrapie should also be considered.

Lumbosacral CSF result		
	Results	Normal values
Specific gravity	1.009	<1.010
Protein g/L	2.7	<0.3
(g/dL)	(0.27)	(<0.03 g/dL)
White cells × 10^9	1.2	<0.01
(× 10^3/μL)	(1.2)	(<0.01)
Lymphocytes %	0	>95
Neutrophils %	57	<5
Macrophages %	43	<5

ii. Examination of CSF should be carried out. A lumbosacral CSF sample collected under local anaesthesia (table) reveals a neutrophilic pleocytosis and elevated protein concentration consistent with a diagnosis of a bacterial infection involving the meninges (lumbosacral CSF results in a ram with focal cerebellar meningitis are shown). A traumatic lesion was ruled out because there was no evidence of intrathecal pathological haemorrhage or xanthochromic change in the CSF.
iii. The ram was treated with intravenous trimethoprim/sulphonamide injection and a single intravenous injection of 1.1 mg/kg dexamethasone.
iv. There was no improvement after 5 days' antibiotic therapy. Necropsy confirmed the presence of a severe suppurative meningitis affecting the ventral pons, caudal cerebellum, and surrounding the medulla, with several Gram-positive coccal type colonies (alpha-haemolytic streptococci). The necropsy findings were suggestive of haematogenous bacterial dissemination with multiple organ involvement consistent with a septicaemic episode(s).

138 i. Replacement of the rectal prolapse and retention with a Buhner suture is not possible, therefore the prolapse is amputated under caudal analgesia. Four stay sutures are placed in quadrants through the skin and both layers of the rectal wall. The prolapsed tissues are then amputated one quarter at a time, placing a continuous suture through the skin and rectal wall just proximal to the stay sutures. This continuous suture effects haemostasis. The end result is not pretty but is effective. Tenesmus was noted occasionally over the next few days immediately before defecation but no further problems were noted.
ii. Various factors may have predisposed to rectal prolapse in this lamb: *ad libitum* concentrates/bloat/excessive body condition; tenesmus resulting from obstructive urolithiasis; mounting behaviour in entire male lambs; coccidiosis.

139 In mid-winter a pedigree Suffolk ewe is found separated from the remainder of 85 ewes due to lamb in 2 weeks. On clinical examination the ewe is very dull and depressed (139) with an elevated rectal temperature (41.0°C (105.8°F)). The mucous membranes are congested. The abdomen is drawn in which contrasts with the normal distension of late gestation. The ewe's vulva is slightly swollen with evidence of a foetid red/

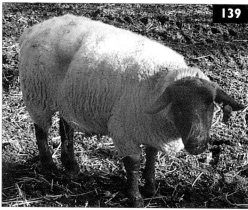

brown fluid discharge. The udder is poorly developed and there is no accumulated colostrum in the glands. The flock is closed with no contiguous sheep flocks.
i. What is your diagnosis?
ii. What further tests could be carried out?
iii. What treatments would you consider?
iv. What control measures could be adopted?

140 During lambing time a sheep client complains that a large number of young lambs have tear staining of the face leading to blindness in some cases. Closer examination reveals conjunctivitis, episceral injection, and corneal ulceration in some lambs (140).
i. What is your diagnosis? (Most likely first)
ii. What treatments would you administer?
iii. What are the consequences of no action/treatment?
iv. What preventive measures could be adopted?

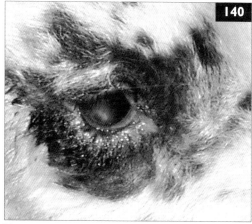

139 i. Abortion/metritis and septicaemia should be considered as the most likely diagnoses. Potential abortifacient agents include: salmonellosis including *Salmonella montevideo*, *S. typhimurium*; *Campylobacter fetus intestinalis*; *Listeria monocytogenes*; *Toxoplasma gondii*; *Chlamydophila abortus* (EAE) but the flock is closed; *Pasteurella* spp.

ii. The abdomen should be carefully balloted to check for fetuses. Transabdominal ultrasound examination of the uterus can be used to check whether the ewe has aborted. Any fetuses and placentae should be sampled for bacteriology and a blood sample collected for EAE and *Toxoplasma* serology. Vaginal and rectal swabs should be collected if there are no products of abortion.

In this case *Salmonella typhimurium* was isolated in pure culture from the vaginal and rectal swabs.

iii. The ewe is injected intravenously with oxytetracycline and ketoprofen.

iv. The farmer should be advised to isolate the ewe for at least 6 weeks, and advised regarding the zoonotic risk from salmonellosis and to adopt strict personal hygiene when handling sick sheep.

In this case the source of infection was traced to a septic tank overflow that was immediately fenced off and the ewes were moved on to another field. Five more ewes aborted over the next 2 days. All ewes in the group were injected with 20 mg/kg long-acting oxytetracycline at this stage. Two more abortions occurred over the next 2 days. No further abortions occurred for 1 week. Five ewes produced autolytic lambs at full term and many of the live lambs were weak. There is circumstantial evidence that the long-acting oxytetracycline injected intramuscularly reduced the number of abortions in this outbreak although this cannot be proven.

140 i. The most likely conditions to consider include: entropion; IKC.

ii. Treatment for entropion involves eversion of the lower eyelid as soon after birth as possible with regular inspection to ensure it remains everted. Topical antibiotic application controls secondary bacterial infection and aids movement of the lower eyelid, thereby reducing the likelihood of inversion. Subcutaneous antibiotic injection (1 mL of procaine penicillin) can be used to evert the lower eyelid. Skin suture(s) can be inserted to evert the lower eyelid but this procedure requires two people; one to restrain the lamb and the other to carefully insert the suture. Eales clip(s) can be inserted in the skin below the lower eyelid to cause eversion and have the advantage of requiring only one operator.

iii. Consequences include rupture of the cornea with herniation of the lens and loss of the eye in neglected cases.

iv. Entropion has a high hereditary component and rams siring affected progeny should be culled.

141 Several 4-month-old lambs experience difficulty in raising themselves to
their feet and have a stilted gait. Lameness was first noted at 6 weeks old. All
lambs have one or both stifle joints
affected. There is little joint effusion
but marked thickening of the joint
capsule (up to 1 cm) which physically
restricts joint excursion. Four of the six
lambs have bilateral carpal swellings
(141a) with associated enlargement of
the prescapular lymph nodes.

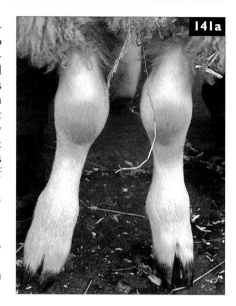

i. What conditions would you consider?
ii. What is the likely cause?
iii. How would you confirm the cause?
iv. What treatment would you administer?
v. What control measure(s) would you
recommend?

142 You are presented with a Greyface ewe 6 days after lambing. The
ewe is dull and depressed with
drooped ears (142). The ewe has a
poor appetite and milk yield as evidenced by her hungry lambs trying
to suck frequently but the ewe walks
away. The rectal temperature is
41.5°C (106.7°F). The mucous membranes are congested. The respiratory rate is increased to 65 breaths
per minute, almost twice the rate of

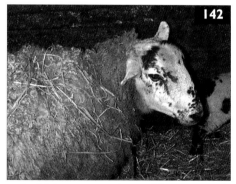

other ewes in this group. The heart rate is 84 beats per minute. No murmur is
audible. Increased wheezes are heard anteroventrally on auscultation of the chest.
There are reduced ruminal contractions. There is evidence of a scant red/brown
discharge on the tail. The udder and milk secretions are normal.
i. What is your diagnosis?
ii. What treatments would you consider?
iii. What preventive measures could be adopted?

141 i. The most likely conditions to consider include: infectious polyarthritis caused by *Erysipelothrix rhusiopathiae*; infectious polyarthritis secondary to tick-born fever; bacterial endocarditis.

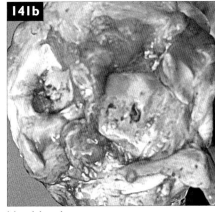

ii. *Streptococcus dysgalactiae* affects lambs within the first 2 weeks of life while *E. rhusiopathiae* tends to affect lambs from 2 weeks old.
iii. Samples of synovial membrane from sacrificed untreated cases are preferable to joint aspirates for bacteriological examination. There is a high prevalence of antibodies to *E. rhusiopathiae* in normal healthy sheep.
iv. Aggressive antibiotic therapy with penicillin during the early stages of infection effects a good cure rate in many *E. rhusiopathiae* infections. However, dead bacteria and white blood cells within the joint induce inflammatory changes including proliferation of the synovial membrane and fibrous thickening of the joint capsule (141b) causing the obvious pain and lameness. Such pathology will not respond to further antibiotic therapy and these lambs should be euthanased for welfare reasons.
v. Vaccination of the dam with effective passive antibody transfer protects lambs from erysipelas.

142 i. The clinical signs indicate toxaemia. The most likely conditions to consider include: pasteurellosis or other bacterial pneumonia; metritis; peritonitis; endocarditis.
ii. There was a marked response within 24 hr to intravenous injection of oxytetracycline and dexamethasone. The ewe was eating well and the rectal temperature was reduced to 40.0°C (104.0°F) the following day; she was then treated with an intramuscular injection of 20% oxytetracycline and recovered well. The fall in rectal temperature after 24 hr could be, in part, attributed to the antipyretic action of dexamethasone. The use of dexamethasone could be questioned but oxytetracycline resistance in ovine pasteurellae is very uncommon, and the rapid treatment response is essential to recover the ewe's appetite and milk yield.
iii. Control measures are limited because a specific diagnosis was not established. The combined pasteurella and clostridial vaccine would seem prudent; the minimal extra annual cost appears good sense.

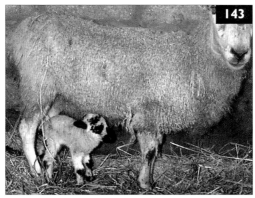

143 A farmer complains that approximately 5% of the ewes in his lowground flock have given birth to very small singleton or twin lambs (approximately 2.5–3.0 kg). The lambs are lively, well fleshed but 2–4 kg lighter than they should be (143). Examination of the dams of three such litters reveals very low BCSs of 1.0–1.5 (scale 1–5), while the majority of ewes in the flock are in good body condition (around 3.0).
i. What condition do you suspect?
ii. What could be done in future years to prevent this problem?

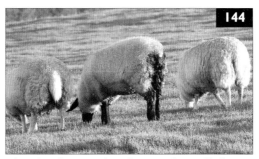

144 i. What procedure has been undertaken on this Suffolk ewe (144)?
ii. When was this procedure undertaken?
iii. Why was this procedure undertaken, and has it been successful?
iv. What other 'mutilation' is often undertaken at the same time?

143 i. The condition may be a chronic debilitating disease affecting the dams, e.g. chronic severe PGE, fasciolosis, Johne's disease, SPA, causing poor placental development and chronic intrauterine growth retardation. Starvation with poor energy supply throughout gestation, may also be a factor.

ii. Very low lamb birthweights can occur when the dam is affected by one of the severe debilitating diseases listed above over a significant period of gestation. Because the nutritional insult persists over a long period of its development, the lamb is well formed but very small. Samples collected from two of the three ewes were positive for paratuberculosis (Johne's disease).

The possible consequences of energy underfeeding during mid-gestation while the placenta is developing cannot be discounted and a review of farm management during early and mid-lactation would be indicated, especially provision of feed during winter storms. The situation could be monitored by regular condition scoring of ewes every month during pregnancy.

Postmortem examination of a representative number of emaciated ewes may help establish an accurate diagnosis of the problem.

144 i. Tail docking using elastrator rings is routinely performed in many sheep flocks. It is a legal requirement that sufficient tail remains after docking to completely cover the sheep's anus and vulva (distal to the caudal skin folds).

ii. Elastrator rings can be used only during the first week in life. Castration with a knife or bloodless castrator (Burdizzo) can be used without an anaesthetic up to 3 months old, for tail docking up to 2 months. Thereafter an anaesthetic is required for tail amputation and castration but it would be very uncommon for these procedures to be undertaken at such a late stage.

iii. Tail docking may limit the extent of faecal contamination of the tail and perineum (but not in this case) thereby reducing the risk from cutaneous myiasis. However, the control of endoparasites, by operating clean grazing systems and/or appropriate use of anthelmintics and pour-on insect growth regulators (e.g. dicyclanil), is much more effective.

iv. The term 'mutilation' (deprivation of an essential part) refers to acute and chronic pain resulting from castration and tail docking. Castration is traditionally performed using elastrator rings at 24 hr old. Such 'mutilation' is difficult to justify because castrated lambs grow more slowly and produce a fatter carcass. However, with an extended interval to slaughter on some farms (up to 1 year) the presence of many ram lambs, which are sexually mature by 6 months, introduces the risk of unwanted pregnancies in ewe lambs and the ewe flock.

145 Two 4-month-old pedigree Charollais lambs in the same flock, which appeared normal for the first 8 weeks of life, now appear unsteady on their legs. The lambs have a lowered head carriage, a wide-based stance, ataxia, and dysmetria but with preservation of strength (145). The pelvic ataxia results in the lambs occasionally falling over, especially when turning quickly.

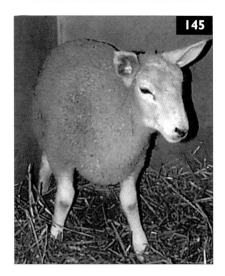

i. What area of the brain could be involved?
ii. What conditions would you consider?
iii. What treatment would you administer?
iv. What control measures could be adopted?

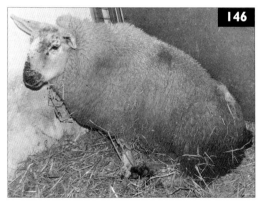

146 In early autumn a client reports that three lambs from a group of 120 weaned homebred sheep have shown pelvic limb weakness since transfer 6 weeks ago to good grazing adjacent to a country park. Examination of a 6-month-old lamb (146) reveals normal thoracic limb function but upper motor neuron signs to the pelvic limbs (increased responses to stimuli and increased patellar reflex).
i. What conditions could cause pelvic limb weakness?
ii. How could your diagnosis be confirmed?
iii. What control measures could be adopted?

145 i. Involvement of the cerebellum would explain the clinical signs. The lambs appeared normal for the first 8 weeks but have deteriorated over the past 2 months, suggesting a developmental abnormality.

ii. The most likely conditions to consider include: cerebellar abiotrophy; cerebellar abscess/focal meningitis. Other conditions could include: delayed swayback; cervical spinal lesion; atlanto-occipital joint infection caused by *Streptococcus dysgalactiae*.

A diagnosis of cerebellar abiotrophy is based upon clinical examination, and lack of intrathecal inflammation (normal CSF parameters).

iii. There is no treatment and the lambs were euthanased for welfare reasons.

At necropsy the cerebellar weight was more than 8% of brain weight indicating no hypoplasia. There was widespread degeneration of Purkinje cells with associated hypocellularity of the granular layer and degeneration of myelin in cerebellar foliae and peduncles. There was widespread loss of Purkinje cells with individual remaining cells being angular and showing condensed, eosinophilic cytoplasm and loss of nuclear detail. There was no evidence of cytoplasmic vacuolation.

iv. Cerebellar abiotrophy is a familial syndrome affecting Charollais sheep. The inherited nature of this metabolic defect stresses the importance of an accurate diagnosis, especially in rams which contribute significantly to the genetic profile of the flock. Affected lambs should be euthanased for welfare reasons and the sire and dam culled.

146 i. The most likely conditions to cause pelvic limb weakness include: sarcocystis (encephalo)myelitis; vertebral body abscess, possibly associated with tick born fever/tick pyaemia; enzootic ataxia/delayed swayback (but not in weaned lambs); trauma of the spinal cord/vertebral column; aberrant gid lesions.

Sarcocystis (encephalo)myelitis is not uncommon, causing pelvic limb paresis in growing lambs, although these clinical features may arise from compressive lesions of the thoracolumbar spinal cord, especially vertebral empyema.

ii. CSF changes in sarcocystis (encephalo)myelitis are nonspecific, with an elevated white cell count and increased eosinophil percentage. Serological testing is unhelpful because high sarcocystis titres are commonly encountered in healthy sheep. Gross postmortem examination may reveal no abnormality and specific diagnosis of sarcocystis infection necessitates immunocytochemical staining of spinal cord sections. Evidence of severe sarcocystis infection can often be observed elsewhere, particularly the myocardium and diaphragm of affected lambs, but is also present in apparently healthy lambs.

iii. Control of sarcocystis infection is based upon breaking the sheep–dog cycle by correct and timely disposal of sheep carcasses and attempting to limit faecal contamination of pastures by dogs.

147 A 6-year-old ewe presents with a history of chronic weight loss (BCS 1.5) while the remainder of sheep in the group are within a range from 3–3.5. The rectal temperature is 39.0°C (102.2°F). The sheep has a reduced appetite. There is no diarrhoea. Auscultation of the chest reveals no abnormalities except a slight increase in heart rate (96 beats per minute). There is considerable abdominal

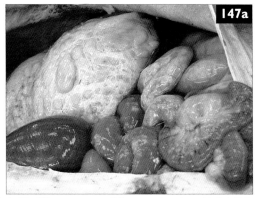

enlargement with an obvious fluid thrill. Ultrasonographic examination (5.0 MHz sector transducer connected to a real-time, B-mode ultrasound machine) reveals dorsal displacement of abdominal viscera by 10–12 cm of fluid. (147a taken at necropsy.)

i. What conditions would you consider?
ii. What further tests would you undertake?
iii. What is your diagnosis and what treatment would you administer?
iv. What is the likely cause?

148 In early autumn your client complains of poor growth in a large group of homebred fat-tening lambs weaned 6 weeks ago. Large numbers of lambs have diarrhoea with heavy fleece contamination (148). The farm is a sheep-only enterprise. An anthelmintic was administered when the lambs scoured in the

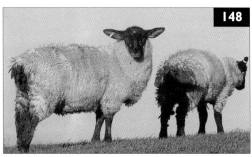

summer, and again 4 and 8 weeks later. The farmer has used a white drench (benzimidazole; group 1) for the past 3 years.

i. What are the possible causes of poor growth in these lambs?
ii. How would you investigate this problem?
iii. What action would you recommend?
iv. What control measures should be introduced?

147 i. The most likely conditions to consider include: adenocarcinoma of the small intestine with transcoelomic spread impairing lymphatic drainage; chronic peritonitis; ascites as a consequence of low serum albumin concentration; subacute fasciolosis, but only one sheep is affected.

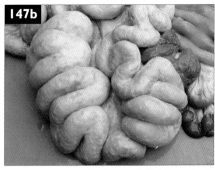

ii. Serum protein and peritoneal fluid analyses should be carried out. In this case, serum protein analysis reveals marginally low albumin but normal globulin concentrations. Peritoneal fluid analysis reveals a modified transudate (protein concentration 34.8 g/L, 3.48 g/dL) with a large number of carcinoma cells on cytospin.

iii. Euthanasia for welfare reasons is indicated after diagnosis of adenocarcinoma of the small intestine. Necropsy reveals loops of fibrosed bowel (147b) with adhesions and transcoelomic tumour deposits on the serosa of the omentum, abdominal wall, liver, and diaphragm.

iv. An association with bracken ingestion has been suggested but this sheep had never had access to bracken.

148 i. The possible causes of poor growth in these lambs include: poor nutrition of the ewe, lamb or both, e.g. overstocking, poor pasture management; PGE; massive larval challenge from mid-summer rise; ineffective anthelmintic treatments (incorrect timing, under-dosing, resistance); cobalt deficiency. Selenium deficiency is much less likely. A combination of these causes may act in this situation.

ii. Faecal egg counts (modified McMaster technique) on pooled equal quantities of faeces collected from eight lambs was 4,200 epg (<400 epg = low, 400–1,000 = moderate, >1,000 epg = high). Ten individual counts are indicated now and 10 days after benzimidazole treatment to establish whether group 1 resistance is present (>85% reduction expected; 40% achieved).

iii. An anthelmintic from a different group should be used. In this case the lambs were treated with levamisole (group 2) and the diarrhoea stopped almost immediately. The farmer was not prepared to pay for serum vitamin B_{12} analyses, however the low unit cost of cobalt sulphate allows inclusion in the anthelmintic drench (15–30 g per 10 L of 1.5% levamisole drench).

iv. In the absence of a clean grazing system (arable crop/cattle/sheep, rotated annually), PGE is controlled by strategic anthelmintic treatments of ewes and lambs and avoidance of larval build-up on pasture. Specific veterinary advice is indicated because such suppressive programmes may be unsustainable.

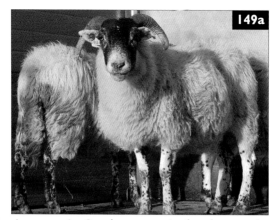

149 While selecting ewes in October to retain for the next breeding season, a sheep client finds 10 of 700 young ewes to be in very poor body condition. You are presented with an emaciated 4-year-old Scottish Blackface ewe typical of this group (149a). The fleece is open and poor. The rectal temperature is normal. The eyes appear sunken which is thought to be largely due to the absence of intra-orbital fat. The mucous membranes appear pale. There is no evidence of diarrhoea.

i. What is your provisional diagnosis? (Most likely first.)
ii. What tests would you undertake?
iii. What action would you recommend?
iv. What control measures could be adopted?

150 In late summer you are presented with six ewes from a group of 95 which are pyrexic (up to 42.0°C (107.6°F)) and appear stiff and reluctant to move. They adopt a roached back stance with the neck extended and the head held lowered. Typically, there is oedema of the face and ears, and some sheep are dyspnoeic. Erosions are present on the lips. There is profuse salivation, and a serous to mucopurulent nasal discharge. There is hyperaemia of the coronary band, and around the muzzle and mouth. The tongue is swollen.

i. What conditions would you consider?
ii. What action would you take?
iii. How is the provisional diagnosis confirmed?

149 i. The most likely conditions to consider include: Johne's disease (para-tuberculosis); subacute fasciolosis; haemonchosis; chronic suppurative pneumonia or other septic focus; poor dentition (molars); intestinal tumour.

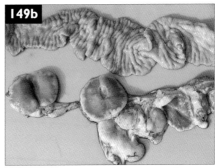

ii. Sheep with advanced Johne's disease have profound hypoalbuminaemia (serum values <15 g/L, <1.5 g/dL; normal range >30 g/L, >3.0 g/dL) and normal globulin concentration, but these protein concentrations may very occasionally be encountered in cases of severe chronic parasitism (chronic inflammatory bowel disease). In chronic fasciolosis and chronic bacterial infection there is hypoalbuminaemia (<25 g/L, <2.5 g/dL) and marked increase in serum globulin concentration (>55 g/L, >5.5 g/dL; normal range <45 g/L, <4.5 g/dL). A faecal sample should be checked for fluke eggs although this may not yet be patent (sedimentation) and strongyle egg counts (modified McMaster technique). Be aware that sheep with Johne's disease may have disproportionately high worm egg counts as a consequence of immune system suppression.

Albumin and globulin values in this ewe are 12.1 g/L (1.21 g/dL) and 40.1 g/L (4.01 g/dL), respectively, consistent with a diagnosis of paratuberculosis.

iii. Necropsy findings in this case included an emaciated carcass with gelatinous atrophy of fat depots. The mesenteric lymph nodes were markedly enlarged (149b). There was thickening of the ileum with prominent ridging. The diagnosis is confirmed after ZN staining of gut sections and lymph nodes demonstrates acid-fast bacteria.

iv. Vaccination has proven successful but is cost effective only when losses due to paratuberculosis exceed 3% per annum.

150 i. The most likely conditions to consider include bluetongue and foot and mouth disease. In foot and mouth disease a larger percentage of the flock would be pyrexic with mouth and foot erosions progressing to ulceration and sloughing of epithelium. There is no facial swelling observed in foot and mouth disease.

Orf is easily distinguished as a proliferative lesion on the gums. Photosensitization may cause swelling of the head and ears in individual sheep.

ii. Bluetongue and foot and mouth disease are notifiable diseases in many countries and suspected cases must be reported immediately to the relevant regulatory authorities.

iii. Diagnosis is confirmed following virus isolation and/or seroconversion to bluetongue virus.

151 A valuable Texel ewe lamb in good body condition (BCS 3.5; scale 1–5) presents with sudden onset knuckling of one pelvic limb. The ewe lamb is bright and alert. The ewe lamb has a unilateral pelvic limb proprioceptive deficit and drags the dorsal hoof wall along the ground and stands with the dorsal surface of the fetlock joint in contact with the ground (**151**). The hock joint is overextended. No other abnor-

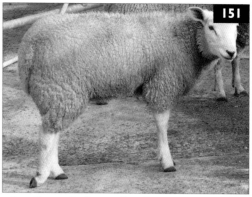

mality is detected on clinical examination. In particular no foot lesion or joint lesion is found to account for the abnormal pelvic limb stance.
i. What conditions would you consider? (Most likely first.)
ii. What treatment(s) would you administer?
iii. What further tests could be undertaken?
iv. What is your advice?

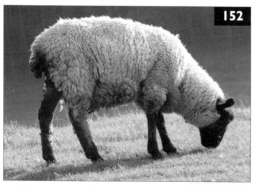

152 When gathering his ewes and lambs for weaning the farmer complains of poor growth rates (18–22 kg) in 5-month-old lambs. The lambs present with a dirty open fleece, and appear pot-bellied with faecal staining of the perineum and tail (**152**).
i. What conditions would you consider? (Most likely first.)
ii. How would you investigate this problem?
iii. What treatment will you administer?
iv. How would you prevent this problem recurring next year?

151 i. The most likely conditions to consider include: peroneal neuropathy following perineural injection of an irritant substance; pelvic limb joint injury/sepsis/arthritis involving the hip or stifle joints; spinal cord lesion such as *Sarcocystis* spp. infection; visna (MVV infection).

Thoracolumbar compressive spinal lesions (T2–L3), such as a vertebral body abscess or extradural abscess, result in bilateral pelvic limb involvement. On questioning the farmer states that the shepherd had given an intramuscular injection of 5 mL of 20% long-acting oxytetracycline into the hindleg 2 days ago because the lamb was inappetant. The shepherd acknowledged that the injection was given into the hindleg muscles rather than into the neck.

ii. The ewe lamb's distal limb was splinted to prevent trauma to the cranial aspect of the fetlock joint and limit contraction of the flexor tendons. The splint was replaced after 10 days and removed after 3 weeks. Alternatively, the distal limb could have been cast. The ewe lamb made a full recovery.

iii. Testing for MVV could be undertaken but visna is unlikely as the ewe lamb is only 5 months old, the flock is closed, has excellent biosecurity, and has remained seronegative for the past 8 years for MVV infection.

iv. Sheep should be injected into the muscles of the neck using aseptic technique.

152 i. The most likely conditions to consider include: trace element deficiency, particularly cobalt deficiency; poor parasite control; overstocking, lack of adequate grazing/supplementary creep feeding. In lowground flocks operating a high input/high output system, including creep feeding from 4 weeks old, it is possible for twin lambs to reach 40 kg by 15–18 weeks old (400 g/day).

ii. Investigations should include faecal worm egg counts and serum B_{12} concentrations. In this case faecal worm egg counts from 10 lambs average 300 strongyle epg (acceptable level). Serum vitamin B_{12} concentrations from six lambs reveal very low concentrations (mean <118 pmol/L, <160 pg/mL) indicating inadequate cobalt status.

iii. Treatment involves immediate injection with vitamin B_{12} and oral administration with cobalt sulphate. Grazing management and parasite control should be reviewed.

iv. The low unit cost of cobalt sulphate allows routine inclusion in anthelmintic drenches (commercial 'SC' preparations, or at inclusion rates of 15–30 g per 10 L of 2.25% benzimadazole or 1.5% levamisole drench). There are reports of increased susceptibility to bacterial infections in cobalt-deficient lambs thus cobalt supplementation should be included at regular intervals. The cost of supplementing the whole flock with oral cobalt sulphate is cheaper than assaying serum vitamin B_{12} estimations, which can be of doubtful significance anyway. Advice about cobalt supplementation in the flock health programme should be included for future years.

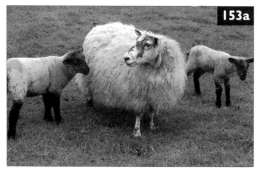

153 An 8-week-old lamb presents in very poor bodily condition after a period of diarrhoea and rapid weight loss. A large number of lambs in this group had profuse diarrhoea 3 weeks ago that was diagnosed as coccidiosis and treated with diclazuril. The lamb is very depressed, dehydrated, and frequently stands over the water trough. The rectal temperature is normal. Its co-twin is healthy and growing well (153a).
i. What conditions would you consider?
ii. How would you confirm your diagnosis?
iii. What is the prognosis for this lamb?
iv. What control measures would you recommend?

154 A 6-month-old lamb presents with a head tilt towards the right side and spontaneous horizontal nystagmus with the fast phase directed towards the left side. There is no circling behaviour. Ventral strabismus (eye drop) is present on the right side. Damage to the right facial nerve has resulted in drooping of the right upper eyelid and drooping of the right ear (154).
i. What conditions would you consider? (Most likely first.)
ii. What is the likely cause?
iii. What treatment would you administer?
iv. What is the prognosis for this case?

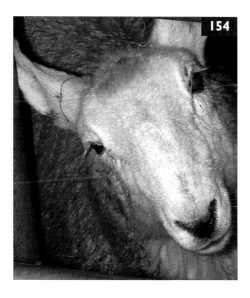

153 i. The most likely conditions to consider include: nephrosis; starvation/rejec-
tion by dam; coccidiosis (incorrectly
drenched or avoided treatment); listeriosis.
ii. Further investigation should include
blood sample anaylsis and faecal examination. In this case laboratory analysis
reveals a markedly elevated BUN concentration (54.2 mmol/L, 151.8 mg/dL;
normal 2–6 mmol/L, 5.6–16.8 mg/dL) and
low serum albumin concentration (20 g/L,
2.0 g/dL; normal >30 g/L, >3.0 g/dL)
consistent with a diagnosis of nephrosis.

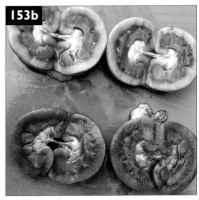

Faecal examination for oocysts and strongyle eggs proves negative.
iii. The prognosis is hopeless and the lamb must be euthanased for welfare
reasons. Necropsy reveals enlarged pale kidneys typical of nephrosis (top in
153b; normal age-matched kidneys below). This provisional diagnosis was
confirmed on histological examination of stained sections.
iv. There are no specific control measures for nephrosis. For future years the
farmer is advised to consider adding decoquinate to the ewe ration during the
last month of gestation and during lactation to both the lamb creep and ewe
ration to control coccidiosis in the lambs.

154 i. The most likely conditions to consider include: peripheral vestibular lesion;
trauma involving the middle ear/facial nerve; listeriosis; acute gid (*Coenurus
cerebralis*); sarcocystosis.
ii. The vestibular system helps the animal maintain orientation in its environment, and the position of the eyes, trunk, and limbs with respect to movements
and positioning of the head. Unilateral peripheral vestibular lesions are commonly associated with otitis media and ascending bacterial infection of the
eustachian tube. There may be evidence of otitis externa and a purulent aural
discharge in some cases but rupture of the tympanic membrane is not a common
route of infection. *Pasteurella* spp., *Streptococcus* spp., and *Arcanobacterium*
spp. have been isolated from infected lesions.
iii. A good treatment response is achieved with 5 consecutive days' treatment
with procaine penicillin, although other antibiotics including oxytetracycline and
trimethoprim/sulphonamide combination can be used.
iv. The prognosis is very good in acute cases. The prognosis is poor in neglected
cases where infection has extended into bone (empyema).

155 A 5-year-old Scottish Blackface ram presents with 4 months' history of bilateral foreleg lameness and stilted gait (155a). The neck is held rigid with the head lowered. The hindlegs are drawn well forward and the ram appears to pirouette on its hindlegs when turning. The ram spends a lot of time in sternal recumbency with the forelimbs extended not flexed as normal. There are skin abrasions over the carpi. There is obvious muscle wastage over the scapulae with prominent spines. The prescapular lymph nodes are not enlarged. There is considerable new bone formation over the lateral aspect of both elbow joints. The extent of elbow joint excursion is greatly reduced and elicits a painful response.

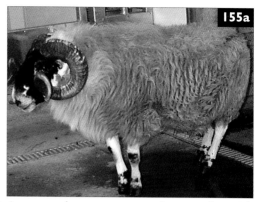

i. What conditions would you consider?
ii. How would you confirm your diagnosis?
iii. What is the prognosis?
iv. What control measures could be adopted?

156 A white-faced sheep grazing a new grass ley presents with swollen oedematous head and ears. Clinical examination reveals lacrimation, and sensitive erythematous nonpigmented skin with oozing of serum (156). The rectal temperature is normal.

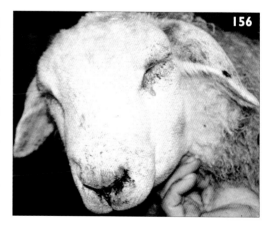

i. What conditions would you consider? (Most likely first)
ii. What are the possible causes?
iii. What treatment would you administer?
iv. What control measures would you introduce?

155 i. The most likely conditions to consider
include: osteoarthritis of the elbow joints
(enthesophyte formation involving the lateral
collateral ligament); polyarthritis.

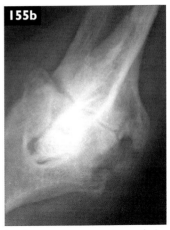

ii. Radiography can be used to confirm the
diagnosis. Oblique radiographs of the elbow
joints reveal considerable enthesophytic reaction
involving the lateral collateral ligament (155b).
iii. Analgesic drugs have no effect on the underlying proliferative bony reaction. The prognosis
is hopeless and the sheep should be culled for
welfare reasons. The farmer was advised that
the sheep would have to be transported to the
local slaughterhouse in a separate compartment
of the trailer.
iv. Rupture of the lateral collateral ligament results from overextension of the
elbow joint when the sheep is incorrectly cast or other traumatic injury. The use
of crates for foot trimming may reduce some risk of injury but little is known
about the aetiology of this under-reported condition.

156 i. The most likely conditions to consider include: photosensitization; bighead
(*Clostridium chauvoei* infection); dog bite to the face or similar wound/cellulitis;
bluetongue.
ii. Photosensitization is most evident in animals with nonpigmented skin. Primary
photosensitization results when an ingested photodynamic agent in the animal's
body (hypericin from St. John's Wort (*Hypericum perforatum*) is often quoted) is
exposed to ultraviolet light causing fluorescence and death of cells in the skin. The
cell necrosis and dermatitis is characteristically most severe in nonpigmented skin.
Secondary (hepatogenous) photosensitization results from the liver's inability to
excrete phylloerythrin, a breakdown product of chlorophyll. In New Zealand
facial eczema is caused by ingestion of the hepatotoxin, sporidesmin, produced by
the saprophytic fungus *Pithomyces chartarum*.
iii. Treatment includes removing the source of photosensitizing agent if identifiable and protecting the animal from direct sunlight by housing. Parenteral
corticosteroids are indicated in the acute erythematous stage of photosensitization to reduce oedema/inflammation. Topical emollients and antimicrobials may
help soften and protect the skin. Systemic antibiotics are indicated in cases of a
secondary bacterial dermatitis.
iv. In the absence of recognized plant species, primary photosensitization occurs
sporadically and there are no specific control measures.

157 You are presented with an 8-week-old Suffolk-cross lamb which has been unable to bear weight on the thoracic limbs (157a) for approximately 1 week. The lamb appeared normal for the first 7 weeks of life. There are no palpable joint swellings or swollen prescapular lymph nodes. There are lower motor neuron signs to the thoracic limbs with reduced reflexes and flaccid paralysis.

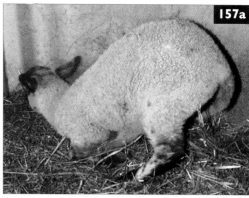

There are upper motor neuron signs to pelvic limbs with increased reflexes and spastic paralysis.
i. Where is the probable site of the lesion?
ii. What type of lesion would you suspect? (Most likely first.)
iii. What further investigations could be undertaken?
iv. What prognosis would you offer?

158 While attending a lame bull on an upland farm in late autumn, you discover your client's dead sheep awaiting collection and disposal (158). Your client has 300 hill Scottish Blackface ewes crossed with the Blueface Leicester ram, and 250 mule ewes mated to Suffolk rams.
i. Are one dead lean ewe and five dead fattening lambs acceptable losses over 2 days?
ii. List the likely causes.
iii. Could such losses be prevented?

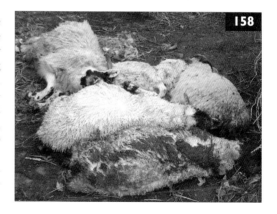

157 i. The probable site of the lesion is between C6 and T2.
ii. The most likely conditions to consider include: vertebral empyema; vertebral body fracture; sarcocystis; delayed swayback.
iii. Lumbosacral CSF analysis is a sensitive and specific test for an inflammatory lesion causing spinal

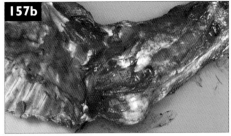

cord compression with an increase in lumbar CSF protein concentration from a normal concentration <0.3 g/L (<0.03 g/dL) to >1.0 g/L (>0.1 g/dL), and frequently >2.0 g/L (>0.2 g/dL). There is little increase in the white cell concentration. Radiographic indentification of vertebral empyema is difficult even with excellent-quality radiographs. Myelography can be performed but is expensive and not without risk.
iv. Compressive spinal cord lesions, whether traumatic or infectious in origin (157b) offer a grave prognosis and euthanasia is indicated for animal welfare reasons.

158 i. Such losses are unacceptable. Annual ewe mortality is quoted at 5%; 70% of these losses occurring in the periparturient period. All lean ewes should have been culled/investigated prior to the start of the breeding season. Lamb losses from birth to sale should be <2%; five dead lambs within a few days is negligent.
ii. The most likely conditions to consider would include: if unvaccinated, pulpy kidney and other clostridial diseases (e.g. black disease); septicaemic pasteurellosis; subacute fasciolosis; acidosis if sudden introduction of concentrates; PGE (especially *Trichostrongylus vitrinus*); tick-transmitted disease although it is late in the season. Cobalt deficiency may play a role in immune system suppression and predisposition to infections.
iii. There must be an immediate review of management practices, including vaccinations, recent flukicide and anthelmintic treatments, and all recent dietary changes.
   A postmortem examination should be carried out on any sheep that died today. Typical clinical findings include: (1) Pulpy kidney: rapid autolysis, pericardial fluid, and glucosuria. (2) Septicaemic pasteurellosis: oedematous lungs, ecchymoses, froth in trachea but changes easily overlooked. (3) Liver damage from migrating immature flukes is readily identifiable. (4) Acidosis: rancid fluid rumen contents ('soupy consistency') containing large amounts of barley, rumen pH value is <5.0 (normal >6.5).
   Faeces samples can be collected for worm egg counts and serum samples for liver enzymes (GLDH) from representative groups of sheep if appropriate.

159 You are presented with a 5-week-old Suffolk-cross lamb which is depressed and unable to follow the ewe. The farmer reports that the lamb has an abnormal gait including walking sideways or backwards. The rectal temperature is 40.0°C (104.4°F). The lamb now presents in lateral recumbency with the thoracic limbs held in rigid extension, flexion of the pelvic limbs, and dorsiflexion of the neck (159a). The lamb is hyperaesthetic to tactile and auditory

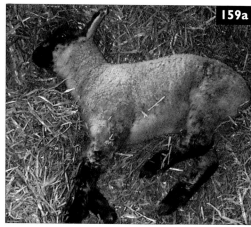

stimuli. Gentle forced movement of the neck is resisted. There is episcleral congestion and dorsomedial strabismus. The menace response is absent. There is no evidence of concurrent bacterial infection of other organ systems such as the limb joints. Intravenous antibiotic injection evokes abnormal vocalization.

i. What conditions would you consider?
ii. How could you confirm your diagnosis?
iii. What treatment(s) would you administer?
iv. What is the prognosis for this lamb?

160 In the autumn a 3-year-old Texel ram presents with a very swollen oedematous head (160). The ram is dull and depressed with a rectal temperature of 41.1°C (106.0°F). The mucous membranes are congested. The submandibular lymph nodes cannot be palpated because of the oedema.

i. What conditions would you consider?
ii. What treatment would you administer?

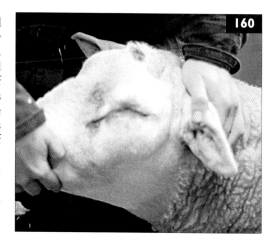

159 i. The most likely conditions to consider include: bacterial meningo-encephalitis; septicaemia; focal symmetrical encephalomalacia; sarcocystosis; PEM; cerebellar abiotrophy.

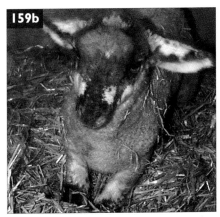

ii. Lumbar CSF collected using a 21-gauge 16 mm hypodermic needle reveals a turbid sample caused by the influx of white cells, and a frothy appearance visible after sample agitation due to the increased protein concentration. Laboratory analysis reveals a 100-fold increase in white cell concentration comprised mainly of neutrophils (neutrophilic pleocytosis) and five-fold increase in protein concentration (1.5 g/L, 0.15 g/dL) indicating a diagnosis of bacterial meningoencephalitis. Culture of lumbar CSF is largely unrewarding and was not done.

iii. Treatment includes high doses of intravenous trimethoprim/sulphonamide and 1.0 mg/kg dexamethasone given on the first day.

iv. The lamb was able to stand the following day (159b) and continued to improve slowly over the next 24 hr and was returned to a small paddock with the ewe on the 4th day.

160 i. The most likely conditions to consider include: bighead (*Clostridium chauveoi* infection); fighting injury wound/cellulitis; photosensitization; bluetongue (but only one sheep is affected and it is almost winter).

ii. The treatment for bighead (*Clostridium chauveoi* infection) is crystalline penicillin is administered intravenously followed by 3–5 days' procaine penicillin at 44,000 IU/kg bid. Some veterinary surgeons may elect to administer dexamethasone at the same time as the first penicillin injection to reduce the facial oedema, however this treatment may not be necessary because the facial oedema does not constrict the airway.

The face was much reduced in size 24 hr later when the ram appeared much brighter and was eating well. The ram appeared normal on the third day of treatment. No further cases of suspected bighead were encountered in this group of rams. The farmer was advised to check on the vaccination status of the group. Suprisingly, farmers often forget to vaccinate their rams and they appear to be part of the flock only during the breeding season.

Ewe number	1	2	3	4	5	6	7	8	9	10
Parity	3	2	2	3	4	3	2	2	5	3
Litter size	1	1	2	2	2	2	3	3	3	3
BCS	3	3.5	3.5	3.5	3	3	3	3	2.0	2.5
Butyrate mmol/L	0.2	0.4	0.4	0.5	**1.1**	**0.9**	**1.1**	**1.5**	**1.9**	**1.6**
(mg/dL)	(2)	(4)	(4)	(5)	**(11)**	**(9)**	**(11)**	**(15)**	**(19)**	**(16)**
BUN mmol/L	2.6	2.9	**2.0**	3.5	2.6	4.5	2.6	3.5	2.4	3.4
(mg/dL)	(7.3)	(8.1)	**(5.6)**	(9.8)	(7.3)	(12.6)	(7.3)	(9.8)	(6.7)	(9.5)
Albumin g/L	34	36	33	**29**	31	34	30	31	**28**	30
(g/dL)	(3.4)	(3.6)	(3.3)	**(2.9)**	(3.1)	(3.4)	(3.0)	(3.1)	**(2.8)**	(3.0)
Globulin g/L	44	46	39	41	45	43	42	42	46	41
(g/dL)	(4.4)	(4.6)	(3.9)	(4.1)	(4.5)	(4.3)	(4.2)	(4.2)	(4.6)	(4.1)

161 A sheep farmer complained of high perinatal lamb mortality in his low-ground flock last year. While the overall flock scanning percentage was 207% at 45–90 days of gestation, the weaning percentage was only 160%, with most lamb losses occurring during the first 3 days of life.

This year the flock was housed 3 weeks ago and penned according to litter size. The sheep are fed *ad libitum* clamp silage and 200 g of mineralized barley (twins and triplets). Serum samples collected 5 weeks before the expected lambing date are ranked according to litter size. Abnormal concentrations are shown in bold text.
i. Which are the important data in the table? (See Russel A (1985) Nutrition of the pregnant ewe. *In Practice*; 7, 23–29 for an excellent review of this subject.)
ii. Why not measure plasma glucose and NEFA concentrations?
iii. Comment upon the protein status of these sheep.
iv. Are mineral (calcium, magnesium, inorganic phosphate) analyses useful in such profiles?

162 In late autumn a client complains that a large number of the 50 ewes mated to a recently purchased Suffolk ram have returned to oestrus.
i. What further information do you require?
ii. What advice would you offer?

161 i. BCSs are fine (target 3–3.5) except for two triplet-bearing ewes. Butyrate concentrations largely reflect energy demands from the developing fetuses with normal values in the two single-bearing ewes 1 and 2 (target for all sheep <0.8 mmol/L, <8 mg/dL), marginal energy deficiency in twin-bearing ewes, and moderate/severe energy deficiency in triplet-bearing ewes; this necessitates nil, 1 MJ and 4–5 MJ/head/day respectively to correct current energy shortfalls. 4 MJ is approximately 300 g of concentrate as fed and costs relatively little.

Following correction of these existing energy shortfalls, continuing demands from the developing fetus(es) will necessitate an extra 3, 5, and 7 MJ/day by the end of gestation in a broadly linear relationship for singles, twin, and triplets respectively to maintain energy balance and optimize lamb birth weights.

ii. Plasma glucose and NEFA analyses are unnecessary because serum butyrate concentration accurately reflects the balance between lipolysis in response to energy deficiency and dietary supply of propionate and glucogenic amino acids.

iii. BUN concentrations are normal. Serum albumin concentrations are to the low end of the normal range but this is a physiological process whereby immuno-globulins are accumulated in colostrum in the udder.

iv. Calcium, magnesium, and inorganic phosphate analyses would be expensive and provide no useful additional information.

162 i. The information required includes how long has the ram been with the ewes, how many ewes have returned to oestrus, and over what period?

ii. Scenario 1. The ram has been with the ewes for 21 days and six of 22 ewes mated during the first 2 days have returned to oestrus. There have been no returns over the past 2 days. While a pregnancy rate of 95% is expected in mature sheep it is not unusual to have a higher return rate if a large number of ewes are mated over a short period, e.g. 22 ewes in 2 days in this case. The ram is left with this group. Another two ewes return by 35 days of the breeding season. At scanning 2 months later only one ewe is found not to be pregnant.

Scenario 2. The ram has been with the ewes for 21 days and 16 of 18 ewes mated during the first 2 days have returned. There have been a further six returns over the next 2 days. A physical examination and semen evaluation are indicated, however the ram must be rested for 5 days to collect a representative ejaculate. The farmer has observed the ram serving normally. The maximum scrotal circum-ference is 32 cm (expected >36 cm). Semen collection from an artificial vagina produces a thin milky-white 1.0 mL sample on two occasions. Sixty percent of the spermatozoa are dead; 25% have detached heads. No white blood cells were observed in the ejaculate. A prebreeding fertility assessment the following year found similar physical and semen characteristics and the ram was culled.

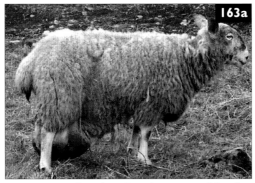

163 In spring you are presented with a Greyface ewe with a large swelling of the ventral caudal abdomen (163a) first noted 2 days ago. The ewe is separated from the other sheep and has a poor appetite. The ewe's BCS is 2.0. The rectal temperature is normal. There is no well defined normal udder tissue. The body wall feels much thinner than normal with abdominal viscera immediately under the oedematous subcutaneous tissue/skin. The ewe is scanned for triplets and is due to lamb in 2 weeks.
i. What is your diagnosis?
ii. What would you recommend?
iii. How can this problem be avoided?

164 You are asked to undertake a post-mortem examination on a 2-year-old sheep maintained at pasture with twin lambs in early summer. The farmer had noted no signs of illness before the sheep was found dead this morning.
i. What conditions causing sudden death would you include in your differential diagnosis list?
ii. Comment upon the gross postmortem findings (164).

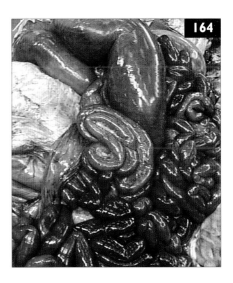

163 i. The clinical appearance is consistent with a diagnosis of rupture of the prepubic tendon. The rupture could contain the gravid uterus, rumen or other abdominal viscera. The diagnosis of contents could be confirmed by ultrasonographic examination.
ii. Serious consideration must be given to immediate euthanasia for welfare reasons. The ewe is inappetent and there is the risk of OPT if her appetite does not improve. There is the increased risk

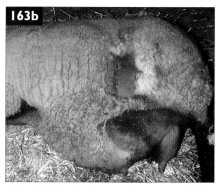

of dystocia and the ewe could never be marketed after lambing. The ewe must be housed and fed a restricted amount of roughage. A truss could be employed to reduce the rupture but this is unlikely to be successful.
iii. There are no effective control measures for ruptured prepubic tendon. The condition occurs sporadically during late gestation associated with multiple fetuses (often three or more) in ewes fed high-roughage diets (often hay and root crops). Affected ewes should be euthanased for welfare reasons. They must not be transported to a slaughterhouse. Dystocia may result due to displacement of the uterus into the rupture site causing lamb malposition/malpresentation. A caesarean operation was necessary to correct dystocia in this Suffolk ewe with a recent ruptured prepubic tendon (163b).

164 i. The most likely conditions to consider include: pasteurellosis or other septicaemic disease; abdominal catastrophe such as volvulus of the abomasum or small intestine; clostridial disease; peracute mastitis; cowped (found stuck in dorsal recumbency and severely bloated).
ii. Postmortem examination reveals necrosis of the whole small intestine containing foetid-smelling material (164). No volvulus is detected. No other abnormalities are found in the carcass. Despite a correct clostridial vaccination history the gimmer appears to have died from a clostridial-like disease. The farmer was advised to review his vaccination technique such that all sheep are indeed vaccinated correctly. The possibility that death resulted from *Clostridium sordellii* infection (not included in all clostridial vaccines) could not be ruled out.

Further tests revealed a profuse growth of *Clostridium perfringens* suggesting that this ewe may not have received a full vaccination course although a positive culture is not conclusive for disease. No further losses were recorded in the ewe flock. The cause of the single death could not be readily explained.

165 A 5-month-old lamb presents with severe (9/10) lameness of the left foreleg of several months' duration. There is extensive muscle atrophy of the leg most noticeable over the spine of the scapula and the left prescapular lymph node is enlarged to five times normal size. The left carpus is firm and swollen but there is no palpable joint effusion. There is reduced joint excursion. The lamb was treated with long-acting oxytetracycline on two occasions, 3 days apart, 1 week after it was first noted lame, but without improvement.

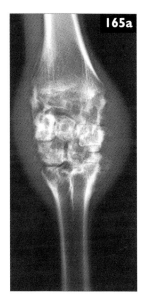

i. What abnormalities are present on the radiograph (165a)?
ii. What is the likely cause?
iii. What action would you take?
iv. Comment upon the management of this sheep.

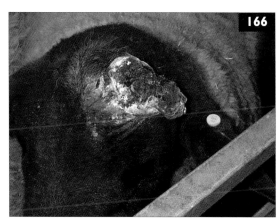

166 You are presented with a ram with a large horny growth in the centre of the poll (166).
i. What is the lesion?
ii. What is the likely cause?
iii. What action would you take?

165 i. There is extensive osteophyte formation and loss of joint spaces involving all carpal joints.

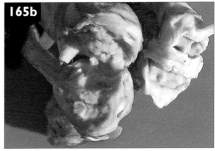

ii. *Erysipelothrix rhusiopathiae* is the most common cause of infectious arthritis in lambs from 2 months old.

iii. While aggressive antibiotic therapy with high doses of penicillin during the early stages of infection effects a good cure rate in many *E. rhusiopathiae* infections, and may render the joints sterile, some infections are not cleared, with the result that progressive and degenerative changes occur within the joint including proliferation of the synovial membrane with elongated branched villi and fibrous tissue thickening of the joint capsule (**165b**). Note in particular the different size and colour of the carpi from this lamb emphasizing the fibrous tissue thickening of the joint capsule and proliferation and hyperaemia of the synovial membrane. The extended interval between detection of lameness and treatment in this case is unacceptable. The extensive joint pathology will not respond to further antibiotic therapy and this lamb must be euthanased for welfare reasons. Vaccination of the dam with effective passive antibody transfer protects lambs from erysipelas.

iv. The welfare of this sheep has obviously been neglected both in the interval to treatment and duration of the severe lameness. Veterinary examination is essential for all lame sheep where the farmer is unsure of the cause and treatment regimen or where the sheep has been treated but remains severely lame 5–7 days afterwards.

166 i. This lesion is a keloid or keratoma.

ii. The cause is keratinization of exuberant granulation tissue often following a fighting injury, and repeated damage to the skin overlying the poll. The role of CPD (orf) virus in the aetiology of keloid has been suggested but not proven.

iii. Such lesions grow slowly and no action is needed. Surgical removal is rarely possible, nor advised, due to the broad base and profuse blood supply. Haemostasis would prove difficult, cautery could be attempted but aggravation of the lesion may lead to further granulation tissue.

Such lesions are frequently troubled by head flies and a pour-on fly repellant should be applied before, and throughout, the fly season. A physical barrier, such as piece of hessian sacking, may be used to cover the lesion but the lesion must be checked regularly for fly strike (cutaneous myiasis). As is the case for all potential severe headfly lesions, the better solution is to house the affected sheep during the summer months.

167 A ewe presents with a history of chronic weight loss (BCS 1.5) when the remainder of the group is within a range of 3–3.5. The rectal temperature is 40.0°C (104.4°F). At rest the ewe is tachypnoeic (40 breaths per minute). Auscultation of the chest reveals no audible lung sounds on the left-hand side of the chest and much reduced heart sounds. Increased audibility of normal heart and lung sounds can be auscultated on the right-hand side of the chest. There is a chronic mastitis with numerous 2–4 cm diameter masses (abscesses?) within the udder. The lambs were weaned 1 month previously.

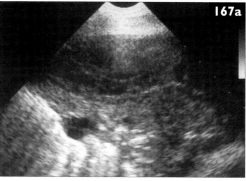

The sonogram (167a) was obtained from the sixth intercostal space 5 cm dorsal to the point of the left elbow using a 5.0 MHz sector transducer connected to a real-time, B-mode ultrasound machine (longitudinal plane, dorsal to the left).
i. Describe the sonogram
ii. What is your diagnosis?
iii. What treatment(s) would you administer?
iv. What is the origin of this condition?

168 You are presented with a one-crop Scottish Blackface ewe which had an assisted lambing 12 hr ago. Severe tenesmus of several hours' duration has caused uterine prolapse which was replaced by shepherd and retained using three mattress sutures but has since re-prolapsed (168).
i. How will you deal with this case?
ii. What are the economic considerations in this situation?

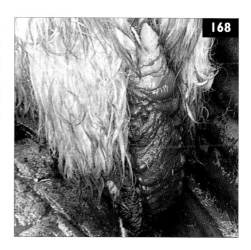

167 i. Normal aerated lung tissue/ visceral pleura reflects sound waves and appears as a hyperechoic (bright white) line moving synchronously with respiration. Examination of the left chest reveals loss of the normal hyperechoic line formed by the visceral pleura, to be replaced by an extensive hypoechoic area with a slightly hyperechoic latticework matrix throughout extending from the chest wall for a

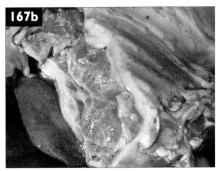

depth of at least 7 cm. The heart is displaced medially by this mass and explains why the heart sounds are poorly audible on the left-hand side of the chest. The hyperechoic line presenting the visceral pleura appears much broader than normal. There is a poorly defined 1.5 cm diameter loculated anechoic area containing hyperechoic dots consistent with an abscess.

ii. The sonographic findings are consistent with a diagnosis of an extensive chronic fibrinous pleurisy of the left chest.

iii. The prognosis is hopeless and the ewe should be euthanased for welfare reasons.

iv. Postmortem examination confirmed the diagnosis of extensive fibrinous pleurisy of the left chest (167b). *Streptococcus dysgalactiae* was isolated from the pleurisy lesions and numerous large abscesses present within the udder parenchyma. It is not unusual to find lung abscesses in cull ewes which also have chronic mastitis.

168 i. A low extradural block should be administered; the first intercoccygeal space is identified by digital palpation during slight vertical movement of the tail. A 25 mm 19-gauge needle is directed at 20° to the tail which is held horizontally. The correct position of the needle is determined by initial twitching of the ewe's tail then lack of resistance to the injection. The injection comprises 1.5 mL of 2% lidocaine (0.5–0.6 mg/kg) and 0.2 mL xylazine 2% (0.07 mg/kg) for a 60 kg ewe. The uterine prolapse is replaced 5–10 minutes after combined sacrococcygeal extradural injection. It is important not to penetrate the vaginal mucosa when inserting the Buhner suture of 5 mm umbilical tape.

The ewe is injected with dexamethasone to reduce perivulval oedema, and procaine penicillin to counter any bacterial infection. NSAIDs, such as ketoprofen or flunixin meglumine, could also have been given for their analgesic properties but extradural xylazine injection provides analgesia for up to 36 hr. The lamb may require supplementary milk for the next few days.

ii. The veterinary fee would be mostly cost of the farm visit and would be approximately 50% of the economic value of a young hefted Scottish Blackface ewe.

169 You are presented with an emaciated ewe (BCS 1.0) with a swollen udder which has developed since weaning 3 months ago (169a). The rectal temperature is normal (39.6°C (103.3°F)). The pulse is increased to 90 beats per minute and the respiratory rate to 45 breaths per minute. There are reduced ruminal sounds. Examination of the udder reveals swelling and hardness of the left gland.

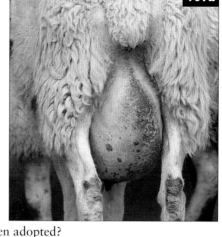

i. What is the likely diagnosis?
ii. Are there any consequences of this condition?
iii. What pathogens could be involved?
iv. What is the prognosis?
v. What control measures could have been adopted?

170 A valuable Blue-faced Leicester ram purchased at auction sale in early autumn was noted to have a 3 cm discrete facial swelling at the base of the ear (170). The ram has been kept at pasture with another 21 rams except for a 6-week service period with 60 Scottish Blackface ewes. A viscous green discharge was noted from the ram's skin lesion on one occasion. No veterinary advice was requested until summer the following year when skin lesions were present in 11 rams. There is no history of illness in the ram stud and each of the rams is in good body condition (median BCS 3.5, range 2.5–4.0; scale 1–5). All breeding stock is retained and fat lambs are sold directly to the slaughter plant.

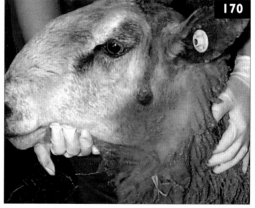

i. What is your diagnosis?
ii. What would you do?

169 i. The most likely conditions to consider include: chronic mastitis occurs sporadically after weaning but lesions are not usually so extensive; exacerbation of udder infection present during previous lactation.
ii. Consequences of udder infection include bacteraemic spread with secondary lung abscesses.
iii. *Arcanobacterium pyogenes* and *Staphylococcus aureus* are the most common isolates.
iv. The udder lesions will not resolve despite antibiotic therapy because of the multiple

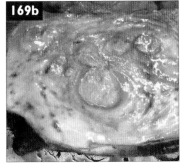

thick-walled abscesses and extensive fibrous tissue reaction (**169b**). Affected ewes cannot be presented at markets because of emaciation and lymphadenopathy. These ewes are unsuitable for breeding stock and must be euthanased for welfare reasons. Postmortem examination revealed the extent of the fibrous tissue reaction and abscessation fully justifying the need to destroy this sheep for welfare reasons.
v. Subcutaneous injection of tilmicosin at weaning has proved successful for the control of postweaning mastitis in ewes but such treatment is considered by farmers to be too expensive.

170 i. The most likely conditions to consider include: CLA (*Corynebacterium pseudotuberculosis*); actinobacillosis. The clinical appearance (parotid lymph node) is typical of CLA.
   C. pseudotuberculosis was isolated from cellulitis lesions on the poll and 2–3 cm thick plaque-like lesions up to 6 cm in diameter in the region of the parotid lymph nodes from 7 of 11 rams. The 22 rams were very valuable and the farmer was not prepared to cull the rams. No CLA had been recognized in ewes at shearing 1 month previously.
ii. The infected ram group should be isolated on pasture that would never be grazed by other sheep. Provided there were no discharging skin lesions these rams could be added to older ewe groups for 5 weeks of the breeding season (also checked daily when keel paint applied). This stud group could be culled on natural wastage over 5 years. Purchased rams should form a new separate stud group mated to young ewes. Strict biosecurity with quarantine of all purchased stock, especially rams, is strongly recommended to prevent introduction of many contagious ovine diseases, including CLA.
   To date (13 years later) no cases of CLA have been identified in the ewe flock despite necropsy of 10–20 thin ewes annually (majority paratuberculosis, occasional SPA case).

171 A five-crop Blackface ewe, scanned for twins, is found isolated and unable to raise itself (171). This group of ewes is at pasture and fed 300 g of cobs plus *ad libitum* big bale grass silage. The ewes are due to lamb in approximately 3 weeks. The ewes had been gathered 2 days ago and vaccinated against the clostridial diseases. The ewes were then moved on to new

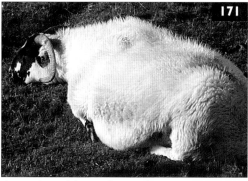

pasture. The ewe is depressed with profound loss of muscle tone. The rectal temperature is normal but the rectum is flaccid and contains a firm ball of faeces. The heart rate is 80 beats per minute. The respiratory rate is 40 breaths per minute with stertorous breathing and a green nasal discharge. There are no cranial nerve deficits. There is ruminal stasis and slight bloat. The udder is poorly developed. There is no mastitis. There is no vulval discharge.

i. What conditions would you consider? (Most likely first.)
ii. How could you confirm your diagnosis?
iii. What treatment(s) would you administer?
iv. What control measures would you recommend?

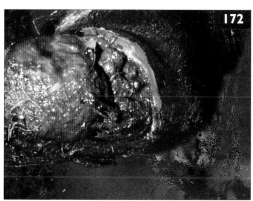

172 A Greyface ewe presents with a large toe fibroma (172).
i. What would you do to correct this problem?
ii. What factors contribute to this condition?
iii. What advice would you offer about future control?

171 i. The most likely conditions to consider include: hypocalcaemia; ovine pregnancy toxaemia; acidosis resulting from carbohydrate overfeed; listeriosis; copper poisoning; sarcocystosis; acute gid; acute pneumonia.

ii. In sheep recumbent due to hypocalcaemia, serum calcium concentrations are <1.0 mmol/L (<4.0 mg/dL). N.B. serum 3-OH butyrate concentrations can be elevated especially if the ewe has been inappetant for more than 12 hr.

iii. There is a rapid response to slow intravenous administration of 30 mL of a 40% calcium borogluconate solution, with eructation and defecation. In this case the ewe was able to regain her feet and join the flock. The response to subcutaneous administration of 60–80 mL of 40% calcium borogluconate solution injected behind the shoulder over the thoracic wall may take up to 4 hr, especially if the solution has not been warmed to body temperature or has been injected at one site only.

iv. Hypocalcaemia is not uncommon in three-crop or older ewes maintained at pasture during late gestation, but can also occur sporadically during early lactation. 'Outbreaks' of hypocalcaemia can result from errors in formulating home-mix rations with incorrect mineral supplementation and inadequate mixing, stress-related events such as dog-worrying, severe weather, gathering for vaccination, when ewes are moved on to good pastures prior to lambing, and within 24 hr of housing.

172 i. A toe fibroma is comprised solely of exuberant granulation tissue without a nerve supply, and therefore can be excised using a 22 scalpel blade level with the sole without the need for analgesia. A pressure bandage is carefully applied over the exposed corium and removed after 3–5 days. The role of cautery (hot disbudding iron) to prevent regrowth of the fibroma is controversial because damage caused to the corium considerably delays epithelialization.

ii. Toe fibromas result from overzealous hoof trimming or virulent footrot, which expose an area of the corium, coupled with misuse of formalin footbaths, which exacerbates granulation tissue formation.

iii. Timely recognition and treatment of virulent footrot is important. Foot trimming of overgrown hoof horn must not damage the sensitive corium. Parenteral procaine penicillin or oxytetracycline is the preferred treatment option for virulent footrot, not footbathing in formalin solutions. If a small area of the corium is damaged the lesion should be sprayed topically with oxytetracycline aerosol and not put through a footbath. If a large area of the corium is exposed a pressure bandage should be applied for 4–5 days and the foot rechecked. Melolin, or similar topical dressing, must be applied directly on to the exposed corium followed by abundant cotton and a pressure bandage. A second pressure bandage may be needed after 3–4 days in some cases.

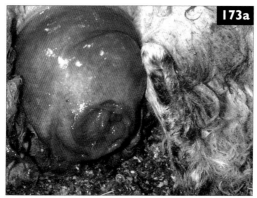

173 You are presented with a twin-bearing Greyface ewe with a vaginal prolapse 2 weeks prior to lambing. There is some contamination of the vaginal mucosa, otherwise the prolapsed tissue appears healthy (173a).
i. How will you deal with this case?
ii. What is the future management of this sheep?

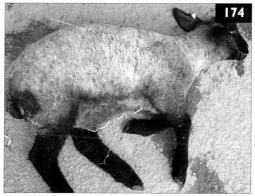

174 A upland farmer in the Scottish Borders reports two lamb deaths (174) and others with diarrhoea in a group of 6-week-old Suffolk-cross lambs on permanent pasture with their dams in late spring.
i. What common conditions would you consider? (Most likely first.)
ii. What tests could be undertaken to support your provisional diagnosis?
iii. What control measures would you recommend?

173 i. The vaginal prolapse is cleaned and replaced under low extradural block in the standing ewe. The first intercoccygeal space is identified by digital palpation during slight vertical movement of the tail, and a 25 mm 19-gauge needle is directed at 20° to the tail which is held horizontally. The correct position of the needle is determined by the lack of resistance to injection of 0.5–0.6 mg/kg of 2% lidocaine and 0.07 mg/kg xylazine (2 mL of 2% lignocaine solution and 0.25 mL of 2% xylazine for an 80 kg ewe).

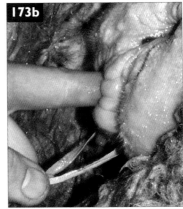

A perivulval Buhner suture of 5 mm umbilical tape is inserted and tied with a opening of at least one finger to allow urination (173b). The suture should be untied after a few days and not delayed until there are signs of first-stage labour. The ewe is treated with procaine penicillin for 3–5 consecutive days.

ii. Risk factors for vaginal prolapse include excessive BCS, housing/lack of exercise, multigravid, high-fibre diets, and lameness; however, these risk factors apply to the majority of sheep which are not affected by this condition. Affected ewes must not be kept for future breeding as recurrence is common.

174 i. The most likely conditions to consider include: nematodiriasis; coccidiosis; pulpy kidney and other clostridial diseases if dams are unvaccinated or there has been failure of passive antibody transfer; pneumonic pasteurellosis; abomasal/intestinal volvulus (single animal only).

ii. Sudden hatching of over-wintered infective third stage larvae (L3) of *Nematodirus battus* after a period of cold weather can cause severe diarrhoea and death in young lambs. Such infestation would explain the diarrhoea in other lambs in the group. Pneumonic pasteurellosis can be confirmed at necropsy; pulpy kidney disease would occur only in lambs from unvaccinated dams. Faecal samples are usually negative for worm eggs in acute nematodiriasis (not yet patent), necropsy reveals catarrhal enteritis and acute inflammation of the small intestine with varying numbers of developing and adult worms.

iii. Control by means of clean grazing with alternate years cattle, crops, and sheep can rarely be practised on upland farms; prophylactic anthelmintic treatment based upon disease risk forecasts is necessary to avoid costly disease outbreaks. If in doubt prophylactic anthelmintic treatment should be used early; such treatment can always be repeated if mis-timed. Anthelmintic resistance is not a concern with *Nematodirus battus* and group 1 (benzimidazole) anthelmintics can be used.

175 The sonogram (175) was obtained in mid-winter using a 5 MHz sector scanner with sector transducer placed in the ventral midline of a 3-year-old ewe. The ewe was presented in very poor condition, inappetant but with abdominal distension. Other recently purchased sheep in the flock are in poor body condition despite free access to good-quality grass silage.

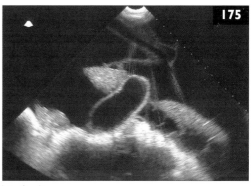

i. Describe the important sonographic findings.
ii. What tests would you undertake?
iii. What causes would you consider?
iv. How would you confirm your diagnosis?
v. What treatment(s) would you administer?
vi. Are there any control measures to recommend?

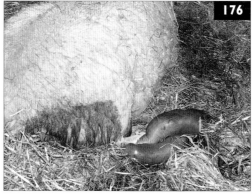

176 You are requested to attend a heavily pregnant ewe with a 'large vaginal prolapse'. The ewe is in lateral recumbency when you arrive and is very dull and unresponsive. The mucous membranes are congested and the heart rate is greatly increased to 130 beats per minute. The prolapse comprises congested loops of small intestine with adherent straw (176).
i. What action would you take?
ii. What control measures would you recommend?

175 i. The large anechoic area, extending for up to 16 cm, represents fluid distension of the abdomen with the liver and omentum displaced dorsally. There are numerous large fibrin tags on the liver capsule, between the omentum, gall bladder, liver lobe, and body wall (inflammatory exudate). The liver is not homogeneous but contains many hyperechoic dots consistent with inflammatory cell accumulations caused by migrating immature flukes.

ii. Abdominocentesis would establish whether the fluid was a transudate or inflammatory exudate (>30 g/L (>3.0 g/dL); more likely as fibrin is present).

iii. The fibrin tags on the liver and to adjacent viscera/body wall would be consistent with severe subacute fasciolosis, although this would indicate late autumn/early winter metacercariae ingestion.

Other conditions to consider include: diffuse peritonitis associated with liver infection (abscessation) although none is apparent; ascites associated with transcoelomic spread of small intestine adenocarcinoma (would contain no fibrin tags); uroperitoneum (has never been reported in the ewe).

iv. Raised GGT and GLDH concentrations are consistent with hepatogenous damage caused by migrating flukes. Changes in albumin and globulin concentrations are not disease specific.

v. The prognosis for this ewe is guarded due to the well established fibrin adhesions. Antibiotic administration and an injection of dexamethasone could be attempted to treat the peritonitis; and diclabendazole given to treat immature fasciolosis.

vi. All sheep in the flock should be treated with triclabendazole immediately and 6 weeks later. Any flukicide treatment in late spring will suffice, including closantel, because all flukes will be mature.

176 i. The prognosis for such cases of evisceration through a vaginal prolapse is hopeless and the ewe must be destroyed immediately. If the ewe is within 4 days of the expected lambing date there is the possibility that the lambs may be viable and an emergency caesarean operation may be indicated after shooting the ewe.

ii. Evisceration of intestines occurs sporadically during the last month of gestation without prior vaginal prolapse or tenesmus. The incidence rarely exceeds 0.5% of sheep at risk. There are no specific control measures. Cases typically arise in multigravid sheep within 1 hr of concentrate feeding. Avoiding excessive ewe BCS (target 3–3.5; scale 1–5) and dividing concentrate feeding into two equal amounts fed in the morning and late afternoon may reduce the risk of postprandial ruminal bloat/abdominal distension. The role of uterine torsion in this condition has also been suggested.

177 A 6-year-old ewe presents in poor bodily condition (BCS 1.5; range 1–5) while the other sheep in the group are in BCS 3–4. The rectal temperature is 39.4°C (102.9°F). The ewe has a good appetite but mastication of food is accompanied by short jerking jaw movements. There is firm swelling involving the left cheek (177a). The left submandibular lymph node is only slightly larger than the contralateral lymph node.
i. What conditions would you consider?
ii. How would you investigate this problem?
iii. What actions/treatments would you recommend?

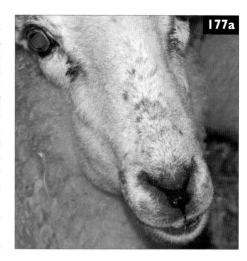

178 A sheep client complains that approximately 25 of 300 lambs (ca. 8%) are very lame on one or more legs. The lameness appears when the lambs are approximately 5–7 days old and have been at pasture for 2–5 days. A typical lamb is bright and alert but reluctant to rise and appears very stiff on the one or more legs (178). The rectal temperature is normal. There is swelling of the joint(s) caused by considerable joint effusion and enlargement of drainage lymph node(s).
i. What conditions would you consider?
ii. What treatment would you administer?
iii. What control measures could you introduce?

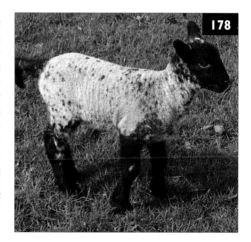

177 i. The most likely conditions to consider include: teeth loss due to periodontal disease; osteomyelitis of the left ramus of the mandible; osteosarcoma of the left ramus of the mandible; actinomycosis.

ii. A mouth gag and torch are essential. Be aware sheep struggle with the mouth gag in place so the shepherd must secure the sheep in the corner of the pen. Typically, the labial margins of the upper cheek

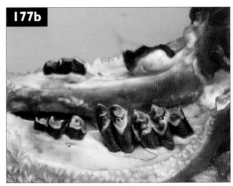

teeth and lingual aspects of the lower cheek teeth are very sharp and longer than normal. In this ewe there is a gap in the lower molar arcade on the left side where a tooth (or teeth) is missing (177b) and this gap contains masticated food material. Digital examination reveals loosened adjacent molar teeth.

iii. Slackening and loss of cheek teeth due to periodontal disease is a common cause of poor body condition in older sheep. Theoretically, removal of loose molar teeth and trimming sharp edges could be undertaken but the welfare implications must be carefully considered. Ewes with poor dentition fatten well when fed a high concentrate diet (up to 1.5 kg/head/day) and this is the best commercial option for the farmer. Care must be exercised to avoid acidosis when ewes are introduced to a high-energy ration.

178 i. The most likely conditions to consider include: *Streptococcus dysgalactiae* polyarthritis; other bacterial pathogens causing polyarthritis.

ii. A recent publication reported 85% of positive bacterial joint cultures yielded *S. dysgalactiae*. Outbreaks of polyarthritis may affect up to 30% of lambs. In addition to the carpus, hock, and stifle joints, infection of the atlanto-occipital joint may cause tetraparesis. Early recognition and treatment are essential. Procaine penicillin is cheap, highly effective, and no resistance problems have been recorded in streptococci. The lambs should be treated with 44,000 IU/kg procaine penicillin injected intramuscularly for at least 5 consecutive days with dexamethasone on day 1. Joint lavage could be undertaken under either alphaxalone/alphadolone- or propofol-induced general anaesthesia but is cost-prohibitive.

iii. *S. dysgalactiae* can survive for weeks in bedding material. Bacteraemia from the upper respiratory tract and ear notching may explain the apparent failure of navel dipping in the control of this problem. The prevalence of polyarthritis caused by *S. dysgalactiae* may justify metaphylactic penicillin injection when lambs are 24–48 hr old, but this is no substitute for good hygiene and husbandry.

179 You need to perform a
caesarean operation on a Texel
ewe to deliver a large single
lamb in posterior presentation.
i. Describe your analgesic regimen for this surgery.
ii. Comment upon the approach
to this case.
iii. Where would you make your
uterine incision (**179a**)?
iv. Would you administer antibiotics?

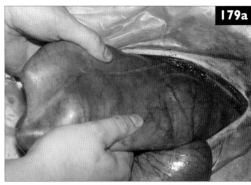

v. What suture material and suture pattern would you use for the uterus,
abdominal wall, and skin?

180 You are presented with a
yearling pedigree Suffolk ram
which has been dull and inappetant for the past 7 days. The
ram has a distended, pear-
shaped abdomen which con-
trasts with the poor appetite.
The ram often adopts a wide
stance with the hindlimbs placed
further back than normal and
the head held lowered. There is
frequent bruxism. The rectal
temperature is normal (39.5°C

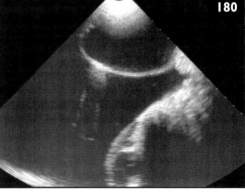

(103.1°F)). The heart rate is increased at 90 beats per minute. The ram shows
abdominal straining but only a few drops of urine rather than a continuous flow
are voided when the ram urinates. The BUN concentration is elevated at 27.8
mmol/L (77.8 mg/dL) (normal range 2–6 mmol/L, 5.6–16.8 mg/dL).
i. Interpret the sonogram obtained of the caudal abdomen (**180**).
ii. What further tests could be undertaken?
iii. What other structure(s) should be checked sonographically?
iv. What action would you recommend?

179 i. The analgesic regimen for caesarean operation includes intravenous injection of NSAID at least 5 minutes before surgery. Distal paravertebral anaesthesia (30 mL of 2% lidocaine) is more easily administered when the sheep is standing.

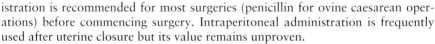

ii. A waterproof sterile fenestrated disposable drape is used but the surgeon is not gloved/gowned because of cost limitations. The approach is via a left flank laporotomy.

iii. A 15 cm long incision is made with scissors in the greater curvature of the uterus (midpoint between surgeon's hands holding lamb's forelegs, note reducing blood vessel diameter approaching the greater curvature) from the level of lamb's fetlocks towards the cervix.

iv. Intramuscular/intravenous antibiotic administration is recommended for most surgeries (penicillin for ovine caesarean operations) before commencing surgery. Intraperitoneal administration is frequently used after uterine closure but its value remains unproven.

v. The uterus is closed with a single layer Connell pattern (inversion suture) using 5 metric chromic catgut on a round-bodied (atraumatic) needle (179b). The abdominal wall is closed using 7 metric chromic catgut with two continuous sutures: peritoneum and internal abdominal oblique muscle, and external abdominal oblique and transversus abdominis muscles. Horizontal mattress sutures of monofilament nylon are placed in the skin (the Ford interlocking pattern is difficult to place in sheep unlike in cattle).

180 i. The bladder is greatly distended and the abdomen is full of free fluid which is likely to be urine leaking across the stretched bladder wall. The bladder is normally within the pelvic canal and is not visualized in normal sheep.

ii. Analysis of fluid for creatinine concentration could be carried out. Abdominocentesis sample:serum ratio of >2:1 indicates uroperitoneum and leakage across the compromised bladder wall.

iii. The right kidney should be examined ultrasonographically via the right sublumbar fossa. An increased renal pelvis to cortex ratio indicates hydronephrosis.

iv. Advanced hydronephrosis is irreversible and the ram must be euthanased for welfare reasons. A tube cystotomy would not be successful due to the renal pathology. Similarly, a subischial urethrostomy, in an attempt to salvage the carcass, would not be successful.

181 In early spring you are presented with a group of 120 Greyface ewes many of which are very uncomfortable and nibble at their flanks and rub themselves against the pen divisions (181a). Some ewes appear in considerable distress and kick at themselves with their hindfeet. The fleece is wet, sticky, and yellow with serum exudation.

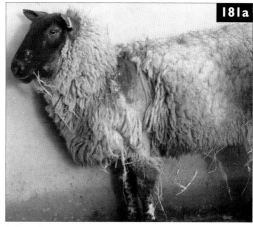

i. What conditions would you consider?
ii. How would you confirm the diagnosis?
iii. What treatment would you administer?
iv. What control measures could be adopted?

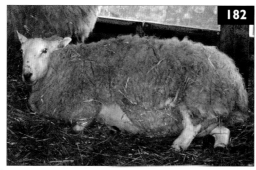

182 During lambing time a primiparous sheep does not come to the feed trough and lies in a corner of the barn. Over the next 2 hr she paws at the ground, frequently sniffing at this area, and alternately lying and standing (182). These periods of increased activity often occur at 15 minutes intervals with abdominal contractions lasting 15–30 s.
i. Is this normal behaviour?
ii. What action would you take?
iii. Comment upon the management of the lambing flock.

181 i. The most likely conditions to consider include: sheep scab mite infestation (*Psoroptes ovis*); louse infestation; keds; severe dermatophilosis.

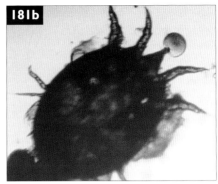

ii. Skin scrapings taken from the periphery of the lesion demonstrate large numbers of mites under ×100 magnification (181b). Lice and keds can be visualized on careful examination of the skin but are not seen in these sheep.

iii. Treatments can include: (1) One injection of moxidectin or doramectin. (2) Two injections of ivermectin, 1 week apart. (3) Organophosphorus dips. (4) Dimpylate- (diazinon), flumethrin-, and propetamphos-containing dips treat and prevent sheep scab, while cypermethrin-containing dips are effective for treatment only.

iv. The reintroduction of compulsory national treatment legislation for sheep scab, revoked in 1993 in the UK, is long overdue for welfare and production reasons. Strict biosecurity and quarantine treatments are essential in sheep flocks to prevent introduction of sheep scab. Sheep scab is uncommon in other European countries. Removal of dipping regulations and emergence of scab in the UK are salutory examples to other countries.

182 i. This is typical first-stage labour which is represented by cervical dilation; it takes 3-6 hr but is more rapid in multiparous ewes. A thick string of mucus is often observed hanging from the vulva. The bouts of straining then occur more frequently, usually every 2–3 minutes. This increased activity coincides with a change in fetal position with extension of the forelimbs. At the end of first-stage labour the cervix is fully dilated. Inspection will reveal no vaginal prolapse which may cause similar behaviour.

ii. The ewe should be left undisturbed and checked if there is no progress within a further 4 hr. Any appearance of fetal extremities at the vulva should be noted, with intervention if the lamb is not delivered within 1 hr.

iii. Housed ewes are unable to isolate themselves from other sheep and frequent disturbances and human interference may interfere with progress of first-stage labour leading to fetal malposture and dystocia. Other ewes frequently claim newborn lambs and are more possessive than the true mother. The establishment of a strong maternal bond is hampered by nearby sheep. The ewe and her lamb(s) should be penned together for the first 24 hr then numbered and turned out into small paddocks of six to ten ewes for a further 1–2 days to ensure bonding.

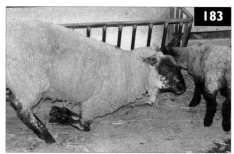

183 A Suffolk-cross primiparous ewe with twin 10-week-old lambs at foot presents with bilateral foreleg weakness with the hindlegs held well forward under the body, propelling the sheep forward with a characteristic bounding gait (183). This sheep often grazes on its knees with consequent hyperkeratosis of overlying skin. This is the only sheep affected from a small flock of 120 ewes. The clinical signs have been noted for approximately 4 weeks. The farmer has found no obvious foot lesions.
i. What conditions would you consider?
ii. How would you confirm your diagnosis?
iii. What treatment(s) would you administer?
iv. What control measures would you recommend?

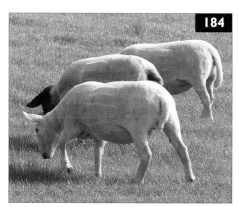

184 i. Comment upon these 18-month-old flock replacements 1 week after shearing (184).
ii. What vaccinations should your client consider around this time?
iii. How should the flock be managed before mating?
iv. How is the flock managed at mating time?

183 i. The most likely conditions to consider include: a spinal lesion, such as vertebral empyema, compressing the brachial intumessence (C6–T2); kangaroo gait; elbow arthritis; virulent footrot or other painful condition affecting both forefeet.

ii. After excluding potential common causes such as footrot, farmers should present sheep suffering from bilateral foreleg weakness for veterinary examination and specific diagnosis. Careful clinical examination should exclude other possible causes of bilateral foreleg locomotor dysfunction. There is no confirmatory diagnosis, and a diagnosis of kangaroo gait should be made with caution.

iii. There is no treatment and affected ewes recover spontaneously after weaning of their lambs. If kangaroo gait is suspected, the ewe and her lambs should be housed and fed appropriately with weaning of the lambs on to creep feeding as soon as practicable.

iv. An appropriate ration for the level of production and available grazing is good husbandry practice and will also help to reduce the possibility of mastitis due to traumatized teats from over sucking. The rare occurrence of kangaroo gait and uncertain aetiology do not justify any specific action.

184 i. These sheep are in excellent condition (BCS 3.5–4; scale 1–5). There is no evidence of faecal staining of the perineum, which may indicate good control of PGE.

ii. Your client should consider vaccination against *Chlamydophila abortus* and *Toxoplasma gondii*. Both vaccines appear expensive but effectively confer lifelong immunity. It is usual to boost clostridial/pasteurella vaccinations before mating and again 6 weeks before due lambing date.

iii. Plunge dipping is often undertaken about 3 weeks after shearing before the peak of the fly season but with enough wool to hold the dip. Dipping controls sheep scab and pediculosis, and offers some protection against headfly and cutaneous myiasis. It is farming tradition to provide good grazing 6 weeks prior to mating in an attempt to improve ovulation rate, implantation rate, and ultimately lambing percentage. However, BCS is more important than a high plane of nutrition so 'flushing' is not needed in these sheep. A vasectomized ram introduced 2 weeks before the mating period, and removed after 1 week, will induce oestrus followed by a shortened oestrous cycle, thereby compacting the mating period and ultimately the lambing period.

iv. One ram is run with 40 ewes as a single group or three rams run with 120 ewes. While the ratio is the same, the latter management system could compensate for a subfertile ram. However, all rams should be palpated by a veterinary surgeon prior to the breeding season to avoid such problems.

185 You are presented with an emaciated 6 year-old Texel-cross ewe with a vague history of pelvic limb lameness (185). The ewe is bright and alert with a normal appetite. The ewe has a unilateral pelvic limb proprioceptive deficit and often drags the dorsal hoof wall along the ground which has caused excessive wear. This ewe was one of 20 ewes purchased from a flock dispersal sale which had contained a large imported Texel flock.

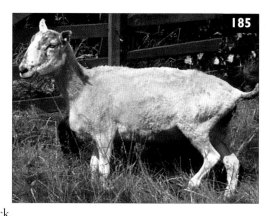

i. What conditions would you consider?
ii. What further tests could be undertaken?
iii. What is your advice?

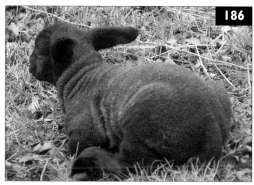

186 Towards the end of lambing time you are presented with two 1-week-old Suffolk lambs with sudden-onset tetraparesis (186). The rectal temperature of each lamb is normal. There are no joint swellings and no swollen lymph nodes. There is evidence of cervical pain and gentle manipulation of the neck is resented. The reflex arcs are increased in all four limbs. The umbilical stump is dry and brittle.
i. What is your diagnosis? (Most likely first.)
ii. How could you confirm your diagnosis?
iii. What treatments would you administer?
iv. What preventive measures could be adopted?

185 i. Unilateral pelvic limb deficits include: joint injury/sepsis/osteoarthritis particularly involving the hip or stifle joints; visna; peroneal neuropathy following perineural injection of an irritant substance; foot lesions such as severe footrot or septic pedal arthritis; spinal cord lesion such as *Sarcocystis* spp. infection.

Thoracolumbar compressive spinal lesions, such as a vertebral body abscess or extradural abscess, result in bilateral pelvic limb involvement.

ii. While seroconversion, detected by AGID test, takes many months to develop, a positive AGID test would be expected if this ewe's emaciated state was the result of MVV infection.

iii. The ewe was euthanased for welfare reasons and visna confirmed by histopathological examination of CNS tissue. The introduction of MVV-infected sheep may not result in overt disease for 8–10 years but afterwards considerable losses can be experienced. Flock screening will indicate the seroprevalence of infection within the flock which commonly exceeds 60% at the stage when clinical evidence of visna and/or maedi first appears.

186 i. The most likely conditions to consider include: *Streptococcus dysgalactiae* infection of the atlanto-occipital joint causing spinal cord compression; muscular dystrophy (white muscle disease); extradural haemorrhage following trauma to C1 to C6; polyarthritis.

ii. A rapid response to dexamethasone and penicillin treatment confirms the diagnosis. Compression of the spinal cord causes an increased lumbar CSF protein concentration (>1.0 g/L, >0.1 g/dL). Muscular dystrophy causes a 10- to 100-fold increase in serum creatine kinase concentration.

iii. Procaine penicillin remains the drug of choice for all streptococcal infections. There is a rapid and dramatic response to intravenous dexamethasone and intramuscular procaine penicillin injections such that both lambs are ambulatory in 3 hr. A further 10 consecutive days' intramuscular injection of procaine penicillin was administered.

iv. Hygiene measures in the lambing shed and ensuring passive antibody transfer often fail to reduce ongoing problems of *S. dysgalactiae* polyarthritis. The shepherd had immersed the lambs' navels in strong veterinary iodine on three occasions within the first 6 hr of life. In this situation it was suggested that the *S. dysgalactiae* bacteraemia arose from either the upper respiratory tract or tonsils because there was no gross evidence of omphalitis. The prevalence of polyarthritis caused by *S. dysgalactiae* may become so high to justify meta-phylactic penicillin injection when the lambs are turned out to pasture with their dam at 24–48 hr old.

187 A pregnant Greyface ewe was noted 2 days ago to be isolated from the remainder of the flock. The ewes are being fed *ad libitum* average-quality big bale silage plus 200 g/head/day of a 16% crude protein concentrate. The flock is due to start lambing in approximately 2 weeks. The ewe is in poorer bodily condition (1.5; scale 1–5) compared to other sheep in the group at a similar stage of pregnancy (2.5–3.0). The ewe is dull and depressed and often stands head-pressing (187a). There is lack of menace response but pupillary light reflexes are normal. The ewe is

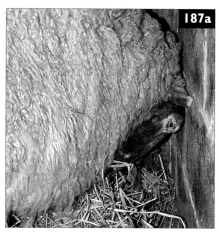

hyperaesthetic to tactile and auditory stimuli. The rectal temperature is normal.
i. What conditions would you consider? (Most likely first.)
ii. How could you confirm your diagnosis?
iii. What treatment(s) would you give?
iv. What control measures could be adopted?

188 An adult ewe presents with 2 weeks' history of moderate to severe shifting leg lameness with obvious effusion of the fetlock, carpal, and hock joints (188). The ewe spends most of her time in sternal recumbency. There are no foot lesions. The ewe has an elevated rectal temperature of 40.5°C (104.9°F) and is in much poorer BCS compared to the remainder of the group (1.5 versus 3.0–4.0, respec-

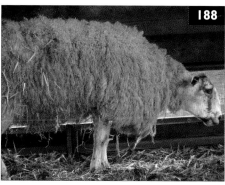

tively). The heart rate is elevated at 120 beats per minute and the respiratory rate is 55 breaths per minute. No abnormal sounds are heard on auscultation of the chest.
i. What conditions would you consider? (Most likely first.)
ii. How could you confirm your diagnosis?
iii. What treatment would you administer?
iv. What action would you recommend?
v. What control measures would you recommend?

187 i. The most likely conditions to consider include: OPT; PEM; listeriosis; acidosis resulting from excess carbohydrates; impending abortion; chronic copper poisoning.

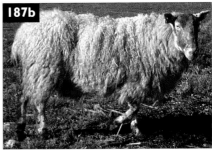

ii. The serum 3-OH butyrate concentration is 4.5 mmol/L (45 mg/dL) (>3.0 mmol/L (>30 mg/dL) is consistent with OPT).
iii. Treatments include a concentrated oral electrolyte and dextrose solution or propylene glycol given *per os* three times daily. Injection with 4 mg dexamethasone promotes appetite and gluconeogenesis (187b) (>16 mg after day 135 of pregnancy will induce abortion which may save the ewe's life). The ewe should be isolated and offered palatable feedstuffs. An elective caesarean operation to remove the fetuses is rarely successful because retained fetal membranes and septic metritis invariably result.
iv. Correct nutrition during gestation is essential especially for multigravid ewes which are at most risk from energy deficiency due to fetal demands. Routine monitoring of late gestation nutrition is strongly recommended and the reader is directed to Dr Angus Russel's article (Russel A (1985) Nutrition of the pregnant ewe. *In Practice*; 7, 23–29) which gives accurate guidelines based upon 3-OH butyrate concentration, fetal number, and ewe bodyweight.

188 i. The most likely conditions to consider include: bacterial endocarditis and associated joint effusions; septic polyarthritis; bluetongue.
ii. Despite the large vegetative lesion(s) on the heart valve(s) in bacterial endocarditis, auscultation often fails to reveal abnormal heart sounds but the heart rate is usually increased. Ultrasound examination of the heart with a 5 MHz sector scanner rarely identifies a classical vegetative lesion. Arthrocentesis would differentiate effusion from sepsis.
iii. Antibiotic therapy with daily penicillin injections can be attempted but the response is poor. Temporary improvement, with reduced joint distension, follows single dexamethasone injection but lameness returns within 4–7 days.
iv. The sheep should be euthanased for welfare reasons. Large vegetative lesions were demonstrated on the tricuspid valve of this ewe.
v. A primary focus of infection is rarely found at necropsy of adult sheep. Bacterial endocarditis in ewes often occurs 2–3 months after lambing; improved hygiene and prompt treatment of metritis may reduce potential bacteraemia and subsequent endocarditis. In lambs bacterial endocarditis is occasionally associated with *Erysipelothrix rhusiopathiae* infection.

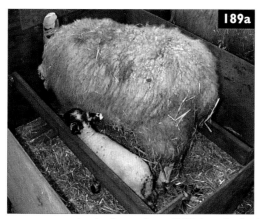

189 i. What management practice is shown here (189a) and why is it undertaken?
ii. How common is this practice?
iii. What other methods are commonly employed?
iv. Comment upon the welfare implication for both the ewe and lamb(s).

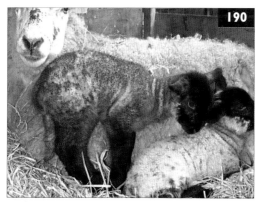

190 i. Comment on the appearance of this 2-day-old twin lamb (190).
ii. What conditions would you consider?
iii. What treatment would you administer?
iv. What action should be taken?
v. How is this problem minimized?

189 i. Use of 'stocks' to foster lamb(s) on to a ewe in an attempt to maximize profitability because hybrid ewes are capable of rearing two lambs.

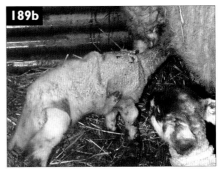

ii. In lowground flocks approximately 10% of ewes produce only one lamb and perinatal mortality ranges from 10–20%. Sixty-five per cent of ewes produce two lambs, and 25% produce three or more lambs. Therefore triplet lambs are used to compensate for single births and high lamb perinatal mortality. The success rate of fostering to weaning is around 60%.

iii. Commonly used methods for cross-fostering include: (1) Rubbing orphan lamb in fetal fluids of newborn single lamb before the ewe licks her own lamb. (2) Fostering lamb by applying the dead lamb's skin (189b). (3) There are many designs of foster crates. The use of a soft rope halter (not baler twine) provides greater freedom and improved comfort for the ewe, provided the halter does not tighten across the bridge of the ewe's nose.

iv. Clean water and good-quality roughage should always be available and concentrates should be fed at least twice daily where the ewe can reach them. There should be adequate clean dry bedding.

190 i. The lamb is dull and hungry with an empty abdomen/abomasum.

ii. The most likely conditions to consider include: failure to suck leading to starvation; dam with mastitis or swollen painful teat or other lesion; early stages of watery mouth disease.

iii. The lamb should be observed to see whether it sucks or is rejected by the ewe. It can be assisted to suck by placing teat in lamb's mouth. If there is no milk present or there is mastitis, the lamb is fed with reconstituted milk replacer (50 mL/kg) and cross-fostered to another ewe.

iv. The lamb should be watched to ensure it is sucking regularly over the next few hours. If it is rejected, the ewe and lambs can be put into a lamb adopter or similar ewe-restraining device until she accepts her lamb.

v. It should be ensured that lambs suck sufficient colostrum within the first 2 hr of life when there is a strong natural drive to suck to survive. It can be checked that lambs have sucked when re-dressing navels at 4–6 hr old.

Ewes and their lambs should be turned out from individual pens when bonded at around 24 hr old into small paddocks with 6–10 ewes and their lambs. Lambs should be mothered-up at least twice daily for the first 2 days. They can be added to larger groups when lambs are 3–4 days old. Ewes must be well fed.

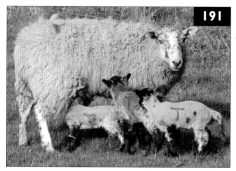

191 Following a pregnancy scanning rate of 207% a client asks your opinion about allowing ewes to rear triplet litters (191). The flock's lamb weaning percentage last year was 160%.
i. Are there increased problems for the ewe rearing triplets?
ii. Are there increased problems for the triplet lambs?
iii. What advice would you offer for next year?

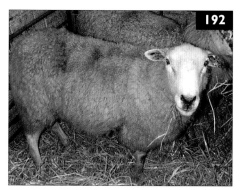

192 A 4-year-old ewe presents in much poorer body condition (BCS 1.5; scale 1–5) compared to others in the flock (BCS 3.0) (192). The ewe is bright and alert and has a normal appetite. The ewe is afebrile (39.6°C (103.3°F)) but tachypnoeic (48 breaths per minute) with an obvious abdominal component to her breathing. Auscultation of the chest reveals widespread wheezes and crackles especially distributed anteroventrally on both sides of the chest. The heart rate is 88 beats per minute.
i. What conditions would you consider? (Most likely first.)
ii. How would you confirm the diagnosis?
iii. What treatment would you administer?
iv. What controls measures could be attempted in this flock?

191 i. Ewes with triplet litters are much more prone to mastitis, particularly gangrenous mastitis, because over-sucking by hungry lambs results in teat sores which become infected, predisposing to mastitis. Ewes are in poorer condition at weaning.
ii. With limited colostrum accumulation in the udder, triplet lambs are more prone to starvation/hypothermia in the immediate postpartum period, and bacterial infection due to reduced passively derived antibody. Lambs fail to grow well due to the fact that the milk supply is divided between three lambs during the first month of life when lambs are almost entirely dependent upon milk. *Ad libitum* creep feed is essential to maintain target growth rates of 300–350 g/day.
iii. In lowground flocks between 20 and 35% of ewes have triplet litters. These ewes are more prone to pregnancy toxaemia and vaginal prolapse; their lambs have a much higher mortality especially if the ewes are not well fed. While some triplet lambs can be cross-fostered on to ewes with singles and replace mortality losses, the remainder should be reared on a fully automatic milk dispenser. A less prolific breed of sheep could be considered or a cross-breeding programme introduced.

192 i. The most likely conditions to consider would include: SPA; chronic suppurative pneumonia; pleuropneumonia/pleural abscess; mediastinal abscess caused by CLA; maedi.
ii. The diagnosis could be confirmed following ultrasonographic examination of the chest. The production of copious clear frothy fluid from nostrils when the ewe's hindquarters are raised (positive wheelbarrow test) is also pathognomic for advanced cases of SPA, but greatly exacerbates any dyspnoea such that affected sheep should be killed immediately afterwards for welfare reasons.
iii. The prognosis for SPA is hopeless and affected sheep must be culled immediately for welfare reasons and to limit further disease spread within the flock.
iv. Control measures include purchase of flock replacements from known SPA-free sources. During winter housing, when the risk of aerosol transmission is greatly increased, sheep should be grouped in age cohorts not upon keel marks (anticipated lambing date) to limit spread of SPA. When sheep are grouped by age, infection acquired by older sheep does not present such a problem because these ewes would be voluntarily culled at the end of their productive lives before significant lung pathology had time to develop. Suspected cases must be isolated immediately and culled as soon as the diagnosis has been established. In endemically infected flocks, it has been recommended that sheep with early SPA lesions can be detected after a period of driving with any exercise-intolerant or dyspnoeic sheep culled at this early stage. There is presently no commercially available serological test for SPA. If there is a high prevalence of SPA in one group of sheep, that group should be culled. In closed flocks, progeny of all clinical cases of SPA should be culled.

193 You are presented with a Greyface ewe with a 6 cm diameter congested fluid-filled loop of intestine protruding from the vulva. The farmer has been unable to deliver an over-sized lamb (absolute fetal over-size) in posterior presentation with bilateral hip flexion (breech presentation). The ewe appears to be in shock (193a).

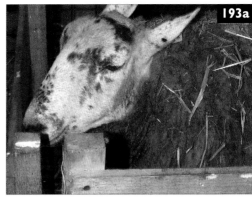

i. What conditions would you consider?
ii. What actions/treatments would you recommend?
iii. What action should the farmer have taken?

194 A 10-week-old lamb has been found with its head pushed against a fence. The lamb is very depressed and stands motionless with the head turned towards the right chest (194). The lamb is in poor bodily condition relative to its twin. The rectal temperature is normal (39.7°C (103.5°F)). There is no menace response in the left eye. The pupillary light reflexes are normal. There are no cranial nerve deficits. There are proprioceptive deficits of the left hindlimb with hyperflexion of the fetlock joint.

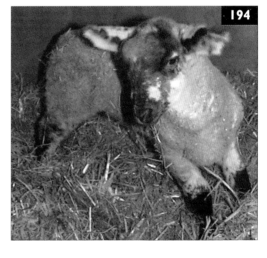

i. What are the possible causes? (Most likely first.)
ii. What is the likely origin?
iii. What treatment would you administer?
iv. What is the prognosis?

193 i. The most likely conditions to consider include: loop of ewe's small intestine through a vaginal tear; schistosoma reflexa lamb; fetal herniated intestines.

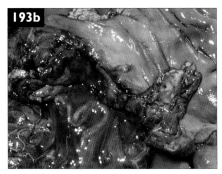

ii. Vaginal examination after intravenous NSAID and sacrococcygeal lidocaine injections reveals several distended loops of small intestine (>4 cm in diameter) extending into the vagina through a vaginal tear. The ewe was euthanased immediately for welfare reasons. A 20 cm tear in the greater curvature of the uterine wall is evident on postmortem examination (193b).

iii. Veterinary attention is essential when the farmer is unable to correct a dystocia. It is very important for the veterinary surgeon to assess the condition of the ewe before investigating the cause of dystocia. Swollen, oedematous vulva and vagina, rapid heart rate, and greatly increased respiratory rate ('panting') with frequent teeth grinding may indicate excessive manual interference.

The prognosis for uterine tears depends upon whether there is contamination of the abdominal cavity, the site of the tear, and whether access can be achieved from a laporotomy incision. If the tear is close to the ovarian end of the uterine horn the prognosis is good.

194 i. The most likely conditions to consider include: cerebral abscess; listeriosis; nephrosis; gid (*Coeneurus cerebralis*); pituitary abscess.

ii. Despite the common occurrence of other bacterial infections in neonatal lambs (polyarthritis, hepatic necrobacillosis, and omphalophlebitis) brain abscesses are rare. It is also unusual to find other evidence of pyogenic disease in lambs with a cerebral abscess except for the almost ubiquitous mild docking and/or castration skin lesions caused by rubber elastrator rings. The lesion more commonly affects one cerebral hemisphere; as a consequence the animal often presents with unilateral, contralateral blindness and proprioceptive deficits, but normal pupillary light reflexes. There are rarely changes in routine haematology values, fibrinogen or serum globulin concentrations. Lumbar CSF analysis reveals a small increase in protein concentration and increased white cell concentration.

iii. The lamb was treated with high doses of procaine penicillin (44,000 IU/kg) administered intramuscularly daily for 7 consecutive days but failed to respond to treatment and was euthanased for welfare reasons. No further cases were observed on this farm (>700 lambs).

iv. The prognosis is hopeless and the sheep should be euthanased.

195 A four-crop Greyface ewe presents in poor body condition (BCS 1.5) when the remainder of flock are 3–3.5 (scale 1–5). The ewe is bright and alert with a normal appetite. The rectal temperature is 39.6°C (103.3°F). The mucous membranes appear normal. At rest the ewe is tachypnoeic (50 breaths per minute) with an obvious abdominal component. Auscultation of the chest

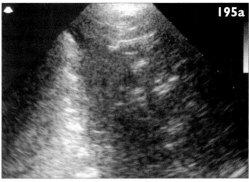

reveals widespread crackles especially distributed anteroventrally on both sides of the chest. The heart rate is 96 beats per minute. No other abnormalities are detected on clinical examination.

i. Interpret the sonogram of the left thorax (sixth intercostal space at the level of the point of the elbow, 5 MHz transducer connected to a sector scanner) (195a; dorsal to the left).

ii. How could you confirm the provisional diagnosis?

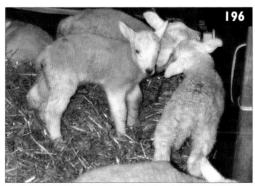

196 A practice client, who has a livery yard and no experience of sheep, telephones to ask your advice on the care and management of 20 orphan lambs (196) she has just purchased at the local livestock market, which she intends to rear in an old stable.

i. List the zoonotic diseases should your client be aware of.

ii. What advice would you give?

iii. What other common diseases should your client be aware of?

195 i. Normal aerated lung tissue, present dorsally (left of sonogram), reflects sound waves and the lung surface (visceral pleura) appears as a hyperechoic (bright white) line. The uniform hypoechoic (darker) area ventrally represents cellular proliferation/infiltration allowing transmission of sound waves. A broad bright line is readily demonstrable where the sound waves transmitted from the probe head pass through the tumour mass then

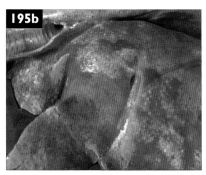

hit aerated lung. This sharply demarcated hypoechoic area is characteristic of the well defined tumours of SPA. Small hyperechoic circles represent small airways.
ii. These sonographic findings are pathognomic for SPA. There is no confirmatory blood test presently available. Copious amounts (50–200 mL) of clear frothy fluid pours from the nostrils of advanced SPA cases when the hindquarters are raised but this 'wheelbarrow test' fails to detect mild or moderate cases. Large sharply defined tumours are revealed at necropsy occupying the ventral margins of the apical and cardiac lung lobes (195b). Occasionally tumours are found in the dorsal areas of the diaphragmatic lung lobe following inhalation of infected cells.

196 i. Potential zoonotic diseases include: cryptosporidiosis; orf; *Escherichia coli*; *Salmonella* spp.
ii. All visitors who handle the lambs should be advised to wear disposable plastic gloves and observe strict personal hygiene.
iii. Orphan lambs are especially susceptible to a wide range of infectious diseases including lamb dysentery, tetanus, and pulpy kidney because of their poor immunoglobulin status. Lambs should be vaccinated against clostridial diseases at 2 weeks old, and again 2 weeks later. Lambs aged 3–7 days are commonly affected by cryptosporidiosis. Abomasal bloat can be a major problem in bottle-reared lambs and many farmers now use automatic milk dispensers with excellent results. Lambs 4–8 weeks of age are commonly affected by coccidiosis (*Eimeria crandallis* or *E. ovinoidalis*). Prevention involves the inclusion of decoquinate in the lamb creep feed or strategic dosing with diclazuril. Respiratory disease is common in housed orphan lambs. Vaccination against pasteurellosis should be considered. Urolithiasis can present problems in intensively reared castrated lambs and special lamb-rearing concentrates should be fed to reduce this possibility. Male lambs should be reared entire wherever possible. Diarrhoea on the fleece will attract blowfly strike later in the season.

197 In mid-spring you are presented with an obtunded North Ronaldsay ewe. The rectal temperature is 38.5°C (101.3°F). The ewe has a sluggish menace response in both eyes. There are no cranial nerve deficits. The mucous membranes are jaundiced (197). Rumen contractions are reduced and the abdomen is shrunken, consistent with inappetance of several days. There is very little udder development and no vulval discharge. The ewe had been fed

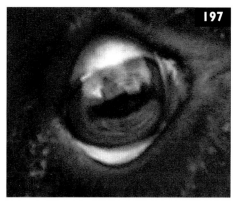

approximately 0.25 kg of cattle concentrate daily for 4 weeks.
i. What conditions would you consider?
ii. Which further tests could be undertaken?
iii. What actions/treatments would you recommend?
iv. What control measures could be taken?

198 A valuable Texel ram presents 8/10 lame for 3 days with a large nonpainful soft flocculent swelling over the cranial aspect of the left carpus (198). The prescapular lymph node is normal sized. There is no disparity in muscle mass covering the scapulae. There is no pain on careful manipulation of the carpus. The rectal temperature is normal and the ram has a good appetite.
i. What conditions would you consider? (Most likely first.)
ii. What further examinations would you carry out?

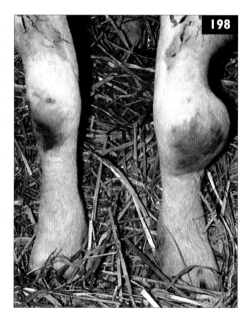

197 i. The most likely conditions to consider include: copper poisoning; fasciolosis; hypocalcaemia; OPT; polioencephalomalacia; plant poisonings including *Rhododendron*.
ii. Serum liver enzyme assays are greatly increased, GGT (480 IU/L; normal <10 IU/L) and AST concentrations (5,560 IU/L; normal <60 IU/L) indicating liver damage. The serum copper concentration is elevated above the normal range (69 mol/L, 439.5 g/dL; normal 9–22 mol/L, 57.33–140.1 g/dL).
iii. The treatment plan was 1.7 mg/kg ammonium tetrathiomolybdate given by slow intravenous infusion on two occasions 2 days apart (or 3.4 mg/kg injected subcutaneously). The ewe was also given 3 L of 5% glucose saline intravenously over the next 6 hr. The ewe was found in extremis 12 hr after first treatment and was euthanased for welfare reasons. At necropsy the kidney copper concentration is massively elevated at 3,900 mol/kg DM (248.4 mg/kg DM) (normal <314 mol/kg DM, <20 mg/kg DM). Liver copper concentrations are usually also elevated but such determinations are not as reliable as kidney copper determination.
iv. Breeds such as the Texel, Soay, and North Ronaldsay are particularly susceptible to copper poisoning. Sheep must not have access to cattle feed and great care must be taken when considering copper supplementation (to control congenital swayback for example). Copper antagonists, such as molybdenum, may be required when susceptible breeds are fed high levels of concentrates (especially when rearing stud rams) despite content not exceeding 15 mg/kg Cu as fed.

198 i. The most likely conditions to consider include: foot abscess plus carpal hygroma; elbow arthritis plus carpal hygroma; infected tendon sheath; septic carpus; fracture of carpal bone.
ii. The lameness is of relatively short duration because there is no appreciable muscle wastage over the left scapula. There is no indication of soft tissue infection of the distal limb because the prescapular lymph node is not enlarged. The carpal swelling is cold, soft, and nonpainful, restricted to the cranial aspect of the carpus, and thereby consistent with a carpal hygroma. This condition, although generally bilateral, is common in rams as a consequence to chronic foot lameness and long periods spent grazing on their knees. Attempted drainage would be cavalier and unjustified because of the risk of introducing infection.

Careful paring of the left foot releases a white line abscess and the ram is sound 3 days later.

Ultrasonographic examination of any soft tissue swellings using a 5 or 7.5 MHz linear scanner could be undertaken if the cause of the lameness had not been determined. Bony changes would not become radiographically apparent for 3–4 weeks.

199 In late autumn, six of 140 7-month-old unvaccinated Scottish Blackface lambs housed for 2 weeks have been found dead over the past 4 days. Some of the lambs had been noted to be very dull and depressed (199), with foul-smelling diarrhoea for 24–36 hr, but died despite treatment with an anthelmintic. The diet comprised only grass nuts for the first week but the barley content was rapidly increased to 90% with the ration now available *ad libitum*.

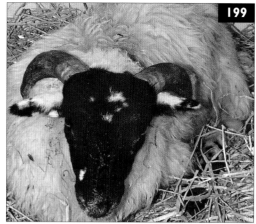

i. What common problems could cause sudden death in these weaned lambs? (Most likely first.)
ii. How could your provisional diagnosis be confirmed?
iii. What treatments would you consider?
iv. What control measures would you recommend?

200 A 4-month-old lamb in a batch of 40 lambs presents at market with severe lameness affecting the right hindleg. Clinical examination reveals considerable muscle wastage over the right hip. The right hock is markedly swollen with thickening of the joint capsule (up to 1 cm) which physically restricts joint excursion. There is no effusion of the hock joint. The popliteal lymph node is not easily palpable. The lamb is euthanased for

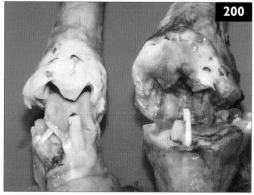

welfare reasons and the hock joints are opened (200).
i. Comment upon the right hock joint.
ii. What is the likely cause of these changes?
iii. Could these changes have occurred during transport?
iv. Was this lamb fit for transport to market?

199 i. Common causes of sudden death in weaned lambs include: acidosis; septicaemic pasteurellosis; pulpy kidney; subacute fasciolosis; PGE (especially *Trichostrongylus vitrinus*).
ii. Postmortem examination should be carried out, including testing urine glucose levels (a useful field test for pulpy kidney) and faecal worm egg counts. In this case postmortem examination of two lambs reveals rancid fluid rumen contents ('soupy consistency') containing large amounts of barley. The rumen pH value is 5.0 (normal >6.5). The remainder of the intestines are fluid filled. There are no significant lung/liver lesions. No glucosuria is detected. Faecal worm egg counts are zero.
iii. Penicillin would be effective against a bacteraemia arising following rumenitis while multivitamin preparations are believed to aid liver function. The role of bicarbonate-spiked intravenous fluids (5–10 mmol/kg (5–10 mEq/kg) bicarbonate in 3 L saline over 3 hr) in recumbent (acidotic?) sheep would be cost-prohibitive in most situations. Alternatively, sodium bicarbonate (10–20 g) and activated charcoal can be given by orogastric tube in 5 L of water. The lambs must be vaccinated against clostridial disease immediately.
iv. The ration should be reduced to 100 g/day immediately and good-quality hay provided. Concentrate feeding can be steadily increased by 50 g/week ensuring that all feed is eaten with 10 minutes. Shredded beet pulp can be included in the ration. The ration is provided *ad libitum* once all sheep are consuming approximately 250 g/head/day.

200 i. There is marked proliferation of the synovial membrane and extensive thickening of the joint capsule due to oedema and fibrosis. There are extensive deep erosions of the articular surfaces with deposits of fibrin/pus in some areas. Note the overall colour of the affected joint – pink due to proliferation and inflammation of the synovia rather than white.
ii. The cause is septic arthritis.
iii. These chronic and severe inflammatory changes are of several months' duration and were certainly not incurred during the journey to market. Radiography could assist determining the chronicity of the joint pathology with osteophyte formation visible after 3–4 weeks.
iv. This lamb was clearly not fit for transport. This lamb should have been presented for veterinary examination either when it was first noted lame or when treatment(s) administered by the farmer failed to effect a cure within 1 week. The veterinary flock health plan should contain clear instruction regarding the common causes of lameness and their treatment, with veterinary examination of all cases which have not responded within 1 week.

201 A farmer complains of severe skin lesions on the muzzle and lips (201a) of approximately 25% of 120 6-month-old lambs, 10–14 days after movement on to pastures containing large numbers of thistles (site of special scientific interest). The skin is oedematous with serous exudation and superficial pus accumulation, has become desiccated, forming hard scabs separated by deep fissures. Careful removal of a scab reveals a deep bed of exuberant granulation tissue. Scab material narrowing the nostrils causes dyspnoea with stertor and abdominal breathing in some lambs.

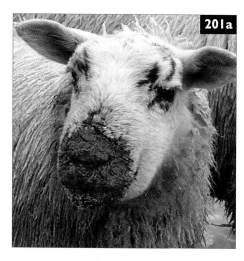

i. What conditions would you consider? (Most likely first.)
ii. What treatments would you administer?
iii. What samples would you collect?
iv. What preventive measures could be considered for next year?

202 In late winter you are presented with a group of housed yearling sheep because they are continually rubbing against pen divisions and abruptly stop eating and nibble at their fleece overlying the dorsal mid-line, causing fleece damage/loss (202).
i. What conditions would you consider?
ii. How would you establish a specific diagnosis?
iii. What treatment would you recommend?
iv. What control measures would you recommend?

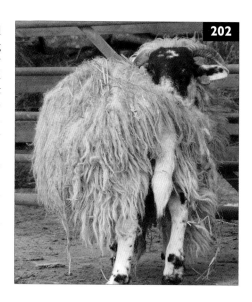

201 i. The most likely conditions to consider include: CPD virus (orf, scabby mouth, contagious ecthyma) and *Dermatophilus congolensis*; CPD; severe dermatophilosis; bluetongue; sheep pox (not in UK).

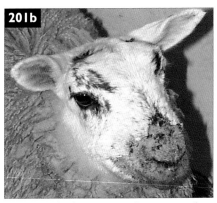

ii. Intramuscular procaine penicillin for 5–7 consecutive days and topical anti-biotic spray should be used to control the superficial secondary bacterial infection (**201b**). There is limited evidence that levamisole (2.5 mg/kg injected subcutaneously every 3–4 days) speeds up remission of orf lesions. Protective clothing and gloves must be worn when handling sheep with orf because of the zoonotic risk. Animals should be removed from this pasture and isolated from the main flock.

iii. CPD virus can be demonstrated by direct electron microscopy of fresh lesions. Bacteriology of the skin lesions is of doubtful benefit.

iv. Orf vaccine must never be used in a clean flock. The timing of vaccination is approximately 6 weeks before the anticipated occurrence of disease. Care must be exercised during handling the live vaccine as it is affected by high temperatures and inactivated by disinfectants.

202 i. The most likely conditions to consider include: heavy infestation with the chewing louse, *Bovicola ovis*; psoroptic mange (sheep scab); both sheep scab and lice infestations; cutaneous myiasis if in summer months.

ii. Lice congregate in colonies on the fleece, therefore a minimum of 10–20 fleece partings per sheep to a depth of 10 cm should be examined using a magnifying glass, with a minimum of 10 sheep examined per group. An average count of more than five lice per fleece parting is generally considered a heavy infestation with *Bovicola ovis*. The slow reproductive capacity of *Bovicola ovis* results in a gradual build-up of louse numbers over several months. Skin scrapings (or clear adhesive tape) at the periphery of any lesions are necessary to detect *Psoroptes ovis* mites.

iii. Louse infestations can be controlled with topical application of high cis cypermethrin or deltamethrin. Infested sheep can also be treated by plunge dipping in a synthetic pyrethroid or organophosphate preparation (availability may vary in certain countries).

iv. Maintenance of a closed flock and effective biosecurity measures will prevent introduction of louse infestations. Annual dipping practices will eliminate this obligatory parasite.

203 A Beltex ram presents with severe lameness (10/10) of the left foreleg of 2 weeks' duration, with marked muscle atrophy over the spine of the scapula and marked enlargement of the left prescapular lymph node. The left fore-foot is swollen with marked widening of the interdigital space. There is loss of hair and thinning of the skin extending all around the coronary band of the medial claw extending 1.5 cm prox-imally with a discharging sinus. The ram was severely lame 6 months ago but eventually improved after 3 months or so.

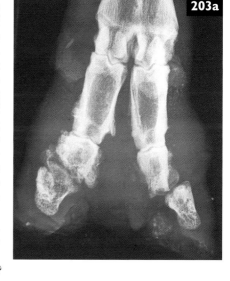

i. What abnormalities are present on the radiograph (203a; medial on the right)?
ii. What is the likely sequence of events?
iii. What action would you take?
iv. Comment upon the management of this sheep.

204 Driving to your next call during the summer you notice a Suffolk sheep in the corner of a field isolated from the others. From a distance it looks as if it may be stuck on its back so you park your car and go across the field to sit it up. The sheep, a 4-month-old lamb, is very dull and depressed and does not run away as you approach (204). There is considerable faecal staining of the

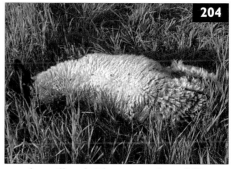

perineum and moist discoloured wool over the tailhead. There are a lot of flies on the fleece; parting the wool reveals a 40 cm wide area of blackened skin with huge numbers of maggots feeding on the surface.
i. What would you do?
ii. How long has this infestation been present?
iii. What husbandry measures must be practised to prevent such infestations?

203 i. There is disarticulation of the medial distal interphalangeal joint. There is extensive oesteophyte formation involving the lateral distal interphalangeal joint, leading to anky-losis. The osteophytic reaction extends to mid P1.

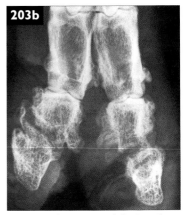

ii. The likely sequence of events is infection of lateral distal interphalangeal joint 6 months ago with eventual ankylosis. More recently, infection of the medial distal interphalangeal joint has resulted in rupture of the collateral ligaments and disarticulation.

iii. Stabilization of the lateral distal inter-phalangeal joint cannot be assured therefore amputation of the medial claw through mid P2 may not be successful. An alter-native is to curette infection and articular cartilage from the medial distal inter-phalangeal joint under intravenous regional anaesthesia and apply a plaster cast for 6 weeks. Analgesics are administered for 5 consecutive days and antibiotics (penicillin) for 3 weeks. Radiographs are taken again at 3 weeks (203b) and 6 weeks to monitor progress.

iv. Digit amputation is inexpensive and effective; curettage and ankylosis of the joint is more often undertaken in rams with higher financial value.

204 i. The owner should be informed that the lamb must be euthanased immediately for welfare reasons. The local authority could be informed of your concerns. Treatment could include NSAID, antibiotic, and dip solution but is hopeless (and ill judged?). Immediate examination of all at-risk sheep should be advised, with treatment for those affected and prophylaxis for all others.

ii. The extent of the lesion and skin reaction suggest infestation for at least 7–10 days but this is only an estimate (and may prove problematic in any legal deliberations).

iii. In the absence of a clean grazing system, control of PGE and faecal staining of the wool relies upon strategically timed anthelmintic treatments which must be part of the veterinary-supervised flock health programme. Where faecal staining of the perineum occurs this wool must be removed ('dagging' or 'crutching'). The synthetic pyrethroids, including high cis cypermethrin, have a much higher human safety margin than the organophosphorus compounds and persist in the fleece for up to 8 weeks after plunge dipping. The insect growth regulator, cyromazine, applied before the risk period, is very effective against blowfly strike for up to 10 weeks. Dicyclanil affords 16 weeks' full body protection against cutaneous myiasis.

205 In attempt to reduce your client's lamb losses you are anxious that all staff employed to assist over the lambing period are familiar with ensuring colostrum intake (205a).
i. What guidelines would you recommend?
ii. What is the most cost-effective method for determining passive antibody transfer?

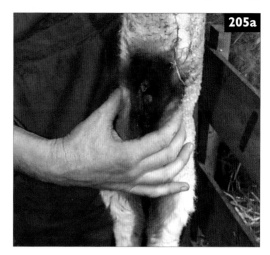

206 A 2-day-old pedigree Texel ram lamb presents with sudden-onset severe respiratory distress and an increased respiratory rate (62 breaths per minute) with a jerky abdominal component during inspiration. The mucous membranes appear normal. The lamb stands with its back arched with its head held lowered and appears in pain. Palpation of the chest reveals concavity of the left chest wall with multiple rib fractures. The lamb dies minutes later (206).
i. What is your diagnosis?
ii. How could this condition arise?
iii. What are the potential consequences?
iv. What treatment would you administer to similar cases?
v. How can this problem be avoided?

205 i. Feed ewes well during pregnancy with BCSs and serum 3-OH butyrate concentrations as guidelines. Lambs must ingest sufficient colostrum (200 mL/kg) during the first 24 hr of life, and 50 mL/kg within the first 2 hr, if not sooner. Colostrum in the lamb's abomasum immediately caudal to the costal arch can readily be detected by gentle transabdominal palpation. This can be undertaken in the standing lamb or after the lamb has been held up by the thoracic limbs. Abdominal distension does occur in watery mouth disease but affected lambs are >24 hr old.

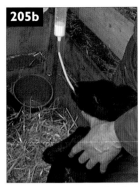

If a ewe has insufficient colostrum, colostrum can be stripped from a ewe with a single lamb or cow colostrum can be used. Pooled colostrum from four to six vaccinated (clostridial diseases) dairy cows can be used (205b). The risk of anaemia induced by feeding bovine colostrum is very low compared to the risk of starvation and bacterial infections. Purchased colostrum supplements are expensive and your client's money is better spent on ewe feed during late gestation to ensure adequate accumulations within the udder.

ii. Total plasma protein concentration determined using a hand-held refracto-meter is the cheapest method to assess passive antibody transfer in lambs more than 24 hr old. The plasma protein concentration for lambs that have not sucked colostrum is <45 g/L (<4.5 g/dL), compared to >65.0 g/L (>6.5 g/dL) for lambs that have sucked appropriate volumes of colostrum.

206 i. Multiple rib fractures at the costochondral junction.
ii. The rib fractures have been caused by the ewe accidentally standing on the lamb's chest while the litter is still confined in a small pen. Head butting injury can occur especially when attempting to foster a lamb on to an unreceptive and aggressive ewe. In newborn lambs the common cause is excessive force used to deliver a large singleton lamb in posterior presentation when rupture of the liver may also result.
iii. Lambs with rib fractures are more prone to neonatal infections, due to delayed/insufficient passive antibody transfer (colostrum ingestion), and to develop pneumonia.
iv. Treatment includes ketoprofen and oxytetracycline for 4 consecutive days to provide analgesia and prevent pneumonia, respectively.
v. Pen size should be a minimum of 1.5 × 1.5 m, preferably larger for triplet litters and ewes >75 kg to reduce overlying. When there is a doubt concerning absolute fetal oversize of valuable pedigree lambs in posterior presentation (especially Suffolk, Texel or North Country Cheviot breeds) it is prudent to deliver these lamb(s) by caesarean operation.

207 During early April you are
presented with a five-crop Greyface ewe which lambed 1 week
ago and is nursing twin lambs.
The ewe is at pasture with 60
other recently lambed sheep
which are being fed 1 kg of 18%
crude protein concentrates per
head per day plus access to clamp
silage in a hopper. The ewe
appears depressed and does not
respond to your approach. The
menace response is present but
slow. There are no cranial nerve
deficits but the ewe is salivating

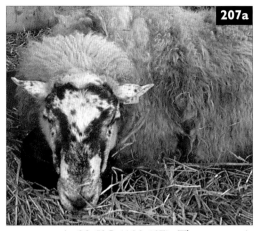

continuously (207a). The rectal temperature is 39.5°C (103.1°F). The rectum is
flaccid and contains a ball of pelleted faeces. The mucous membranes appear
normal. The heart rate is 60 beats per minute. The respiratory rate is 18 breaths per
minute. There is reduced ruminal movement with mainly gaseous sounds. There is
reduced rumen fill. There is no mastitis. There is no vulval discharge or swelling.
i. What conditions would you consider? (Most likely first.)
ii. What treatment would you administer?
iii. What control measures would you recommend?

208 A Suffolk ram presents with
a very large (15 cm diameter)
brisket sore (208).
i. What is the likely cause?
ii. What treatment would you
recommend?
iii. What alternative husbandry
practices would you recommend?

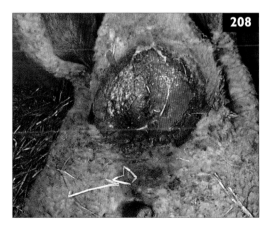

207 i. The most likely conditions to consider include: hypocalcaemia; acidosis resulting from carbohydrate overfeed; mastitis; metritis; pneumonia; listeriosis; copper poisoning; hypomagnesaemia.

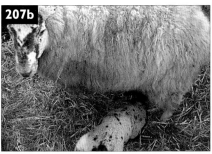

ii. The provisional diagnosis of hypocalcaemia is proven correct after the rapid response to slow intravenous administration of 40 mL of a 40% calcium borogluconate solution. Eructation was observed during the intravenous calcium administration. Characteristically, the ewe stood within 5 minutes of intravenous injection, urinated, and rejoined her lambs (207b). While it has become standard practice to also administer approximately 40 mL of a 40% calcium borogluconate solution subcutaneously the usefulness of this 'depot injection' has never been proven.

iii. There are no specific control measures. Hypocalcaemia is more common in three-crop or older ewes maintained at pasture during late gestation but also occurs sporadically during early lactation. Hypocalcaemia should always be considered in ewes which show depression/recumbency during late gestation and early lactation. In sheep recumbent due to hypocalcaemia, serum calcium concentrations are <1.0 mmol/L (<4.0 mg/dL).

208 i. Brisket sores most commonly arise from poorly fitting harnesses used to hold marker crayons during the mating period. Lesions may also arise from prolonged sternal recumbency caused by severe lameness.

ii. These lesions prove very difficult to treat and never fully heal. Prevention is paramount. Topical antibiotics will limit secondary bacterial infection. These animals are best kept at pasture to prevent straw adhering to the granulating surface. Check constantly for cutaneous myiasis but this is a rare site for strike.

iii. Keel marks are used as a management aid to optimize limited accommodation over the lambing period. In most situations it is not necessary to use keel paint for the first 7 days or so of the mating period when 60–80% of the ewes are served. Thereafter keel paint can be applied to identify the ewes mated after 7 days (housed later). Returns after one oestrous cycle can be identified by a colour change at 14 days. If a large number of ewes are identified as returns (>20%) then the fertility of the ram(s) should be questioned. Alternatives to harnesses include keel paint applied daily during the service period to the fleece immediately cranial to the prepuce when the rams are fed. This method has the advantage that the ram must fully mount the ewe to mark the ewe's tailhead, and the extra feeding helps maintain body condition of the rams during the breeding season.

209 A Suffolk ram presents with severe lameness (10/10) of the left pelvic limb and marked muscle atrophy over the hip region. The left hindfoot is swollen with marked widening of the interdigital space. There is loss of hair and thinning of the skin extending all around the coronary band of the medial claw extending proximally for 1.5 cm with a discharging sinus (209a).
i. What conditions would you consider?
ii. How would you confirm your diagnosis?
iii. What treatment would you recommend?

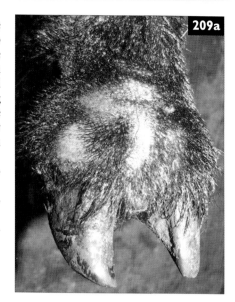

210 A 2-month-old twin Scottish Blackface lamb is bright and alert but unable to use its pelvic limbs and adopts a dog-sitting position. The lamb has exhibited no abnormalities until noted by the farmer 1 week ago. The lamb was treated for 7 consecutive days with procaine penicillin but without improvement. There are no significant lesions apart from those involving the vertebral column/spinal canal noted at necropsy (210).
i. What is this lesion noted at necropsy?
ii. What is the origin of this problem?
iii. What treatments could have been administered?
iv. How can this condition be prevented?

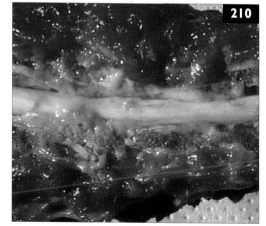

209 i. The most likely conditions to consider include: septic pedal arthritis; interdigital infection; white line abscess extending to the coronary band.

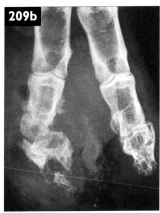

ii. The combination of widening of the interdigital space and a discharging sinus above the coronary band on the abaxial aspect of the hoof wall is consistent with septic pedal arthritis. The diagnosis could be confirmed by radiography (209b) but this is cost-prohibitive in most practical situations. Arthrocentesis is rarely undertaken because there is only a small amount of inspissated pus present within the joint.

iii. Digital amputation is recommended. Flunixin is injected intravenously before surgery. A strong rubber band tourniquet is applied below the hock, and 5–7 mL of 2% lidocaine solution is injected into the superficial vein running on the craniolateral aspect of the third metatarsal bone (recurrent metatarsal vein) (intravenous regional anaesthesia). Analgesia is achieved within 2 minutes. The interdigital skin is incised as close to the infected tissue as possible and the incision extended for the full length of the interdigital space to a depth of 1.5 cm. A length of embryotomy wire is introduced into the incision and the medial digit removed at the level of mid P2. A melolin dressing is applied to the wound and a pressure bandage applied. Analgesics and antibiotics are administered for 4 more days. The dressing is changed after 4 days.

210 i. This lesion is vertebral empyema.

ii. The infection has originated from a bacteraemia with initial localization in a vertebral body articular facet with spread to the vertebral body and spinal canal. On many hill farms vertebral body abscessation and polyarthritis are not uncommon sequelae to tick-borne fever and tick bite pyaemia.

iii. Treatment of vertebral empyema with antibiotics is never successful because of the extensive bone destruction present when clinical signs appear (208). The lamb must be euthanased for welfare reasons once a definitive diagnosis has been established by demonstrating a more than four-fold increase in lumbar CSF protein concentration (normal <0.3 g/L, <0.03 g/dL). Culture of lumbar CSF is unrewarding because the swelling and infection are extradural. Plain radiographs often fail to reveal the bone lysis caused by the empyema. Myelography will clearly identify the site of the lesion but is costly and requires general anaesthesia

iv. The condition occurs sporadically (for example one case per 500 lambs) unless caused by tick-borne fever and tick bite pyaemia.

211 You are presented with a 4-year-old Texel ram that the shepherd complains has a swollen cheek and is in much poorer bodily condition than the other sheep in the group (211a). On clinical examination the ram is bright and alert but is in poor bodily condition (BCS 1.5; scale 1–5) while the other sheep in the group are in condition 3.5–4. The rectal temperature is 39.8°C (103.6°F). The left horizontal ramus of the mandible is grossly swollen. The left submandibular

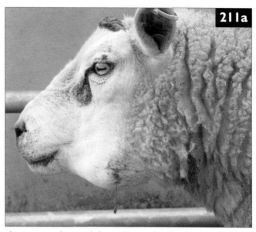

lymph node is slightly larger than the contralateral lymph node. Examination of the mouth with a gag is greatly resented by the ram but reveals a large firm granulomatous mass beneath the tongue occupying almost the complete ventral aspect of the buccal cavity. Further examination of the lesion proves difficult.
i. What conditions would you consider?
ii. Which further tests could be undertaken?
iii. What actions/treatments would you recommend?

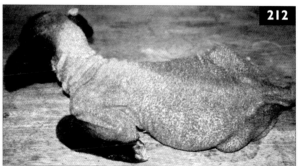

212 A 3-day-old Suffolk male lamb presents in sternal recumbency with increasing abdominal distension and mild colic (212). The lamb was bright and alert for the first 2 days of life but has since stopped sucking its dam.
i. What conditions would you consider?
ii. What action would you take?

211 i. The most likely conditions to consider include: squamous cell or other tumour mass; actinomycosis; foreign body and associated granulomatous lesion; tooth root abscess.

ii. Examination of the mass proved very difficult; a more detailed examination could be performed under general anaesthesia.

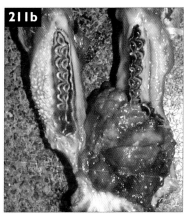

The ram was anaesthetized with pentobarbital (20 mg/kg) injected intravenously (no alternative licensed general anaesthetic is available in many countries). The mass appeared to originate from the buccal mucosa of the left premolar area and extended for approximately 8–10 cm caudally and was approximately 3 cm deep. The premolars were loose within the sockets. The mass appeared to have a broad base and bled readily upon digital examination. Histopathological examination confirmed the mass to be a fibrosarcoma (**211b**). Oral tumours are uncommon in sheep.

iii. Removal was not possible, and this fact plus loosening of the premolars indicated that the ram should be euthanased for welfare reasons.

212 i. The most likely conditions to consider include: atresia ani/coli; watery mouth disease; uroperitoneum resulting from constriction of the urethra by the elastrator ring placed around the penis at the neck of the scrotum; abomasal bloat or volvulus.

ii. Clinical examination reveals that the lamb has no anus. A bulge is present under the skin where the anus should be.

A caudal block is administered using 0.3 mL 2% lidocaine solution at the first intercoccygeal or sacrococcygeal site using a 23-gauge 16 mm needle. A stab incision is made over the skin bulge with a 15T surgical blade. Incision of the skin bulge releases a large amount of gas and mucoid material. Pelvic limb paresis was noted in this case approximately 10 minutes after extradural injection as the result of slight lidocaine overdose but normal limb strength returned after 2 hr. The farmer was advised to gently insert a thermometer into the rectum twice daily for the next week to prevent stricture of the incision site. The lamb was treated with intramuscular procaine penicillin once daily for 5 consecutive days. The lamb made an uneventful recovery.

213 A six year-old Texel ram presents with 6/10 lameness affecting the left hindleg (213a). The onset of lameness was insidious but the severity has increased over the past 3 months and the ram spends much more time than normal lying down. The ram is bright and alert with a good appetite. There is normal anal and bladder tone. There is considerable muscle atrophy over the left hip.

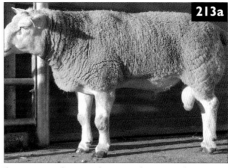

Careful palpation of the left hindleg fails to reveal any abnormality involving, or distal to, the left stifle joint.
i. What conditions would you consider?
ii. How could you confirm your diagnosis?
iii. What action would you take?

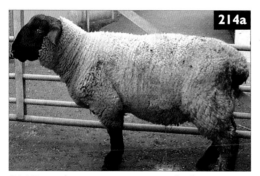
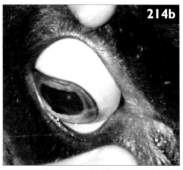

214 In early autumn you are asked to examine some pedigree Suffolk rams which are in very poor condition (BCS 1.5, scale 1–5). The rams, purchased as yearlings, are grazing permanent pasture and were treated with albendazole (group 1 – benzimidazoles) in late spring and again 2 months later. Many rams have diarrhoea with considerable faecal staining of the perineum. The rams are bright and alert but in much poorer bodily condition than expected. A ram purchased last autumn is especially thin (BCS 1.0) and depressed (214a) with pale mucous membranes (214b) and slight submandibular oedema. The heart rate and respiratory rates are increased.
i. What conditions would you consider?
ii. What tests would you undertake?
iii. What control measures would you adopt?

213 i. The most likely conditions to consider include: severe hip arthritis; septic hip joint; visna; femoral fracture involving the greater trochanter; pelvic fracture involving the acetabulum. There is no evidence of hip dislocation (upward and cranial displacement). The pelvis appears symmetrical. A diagnosis of hip arthritis is based upon insidious onset with resultant chronic severe lameness originating above the stifle but not involving the pelvis.

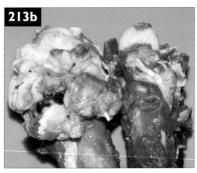

ii. The overlying muscle masses and periarticular reaction present considerable problems with interpretation of ultrasound images of the hip joint. Radiography necessitates dorsal recumbency and either deep sedation or general anaesthesia. General anaesthesia was achieved in this ram with 20 mg/kg pentobarbital injected intravenously over 20 s. There is loss of the acetabular rim with an indistinct femoral head resulting from complete loss of the normal joint structure.

iii. The ram was euthanased immediately. Necropsy revealed extensive fibrous tissue reaction surrounding the joint with complete erosion of articular surfaces (213b). The veterinary flock health plan should contain clear instruction regarding the common causes of lameness and their treatment with veterinary examination of all cases that have not recovered within 1 week.

214 i. The most likely conditions to consider include: PGE, including haemonchosis (possible anthelmintic resistance); acute fasciolosis; poor nutrition, e.g. overstocking, poor pasture management.

ii. Further tests include collection of faeces samples for worm egg count. Faeces samples collected from the anaemic ram reveal an egg count of 42,000 epg. Approximately equal quantities of faeces collected from eight other rams and pooled reveal 6,200 epg (<400 epg = low, 400–1,000 = moderate, >1,000 epg = high).

A diagnosis of PGE, most probably haemonchosis, was based upon the clinical signs of anaemia, severe weight loss, and a very high worm count in the severely affected ram, and supported by the high pooled faecal sample from the group. All the rams were treated with ivermectin (group 3 anthelmintic) and the farmer was advised regarding future worm control for the whole flock.

iii. Control measures include strict quarantine of all purchased stock and treatment with both group 2 (mainly levamisole) and 3 (avermectin and milbemycin) anthelmintics upon arrival. After 48 hr, treated sheep can then be turned out to pasture previously grazed by sheep to dilute out any eggs from surviving (resistant) worms. Accurate dosage for the heaviest sheep in the group is essential.

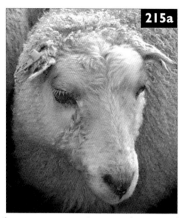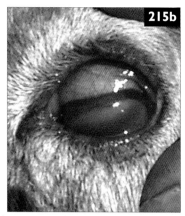

215 After severe weather conditions of driving wind and snow a shepherd complains that a large number of heavily pregnant ewes on the hill have suddenly become blind. The ewes are markedly photophobic with blepharospasm and epiphora with tear staining of the cheeks (215a). Clinical examination reveals pronounced conjunctivitis and keratitis (215b). In some eyes there is also corneal ulceration more clearly observed after fluorescein dye strips have been placed in contact with the eye.
i. What conditions would you consider?
ii. What treatments would you recommend?
iii. What action would you recommend?

216 A yearling pedigree Suffolk ram presents with colic of 6 hr duration. The ram shows abdominal straining but only a few drops of urine rather than a continuous flow are voided. The urine is slightly blood tinged. There are no calculi on the preputial hairs. There is frequent bruxism (teeth grinding). The rectal temperature is normal (39.5°C (103.1°F)). The heart rate is increased to 90 beats per minute. The mucous membranes are normal. Auscultation of the chest fails to reveal any abnormalities. There are reduced rumen sounds.
i. What conditions would you consider? (Most likely first.)
ii. What action would you take?
iii. What further investigation could be undertaken?
iv. What sequelae could result in neglected cases?
v. What control measures would you recommend?

215 i. The most likely conditions to consider include: IKC; periorbital eczema.

ii. The two common causal organisms of IKC, *Mycoplasma conjunctivae* and *Chlamydia psittaci*, are each susceptible to wide range of antibiotics including oxytetracycline. Topical oxytetracycline ophthalmic ointment or powder can be applied twice daily for 3 days; powder adheres to the moist conjunctivae (**213b**) whereas ointment tends to slip off the cornea especially when the contents of the tube are cold. In addition, ewes with bilateral corneal lesions should be injected with long-acting oxytetracycline.

iii. Ewes with impaired vision in both eyes must be housed, thereby ensuring adequate feeding to prevent OPT. The ewes are markedly photophobic and housing will prevent direct exposure to strong sunlight especially when there is snow cover on the ground. Confinement also prevents deaths from misadventure. Ewes should be taken off exposed hill ground when storms are forecast but this is not always possible. Occasionally, outbreaks of IKC occur associated with concentrate/roughage feeding when space allowance should be increased.

216 i. The most likely conditions to consider include: obstructive urolithiasis; cystitis; bloat.

ii. The ram should be cast on to its hindquarters and the penis extruded by straightening the sigmoid flexure. A calculus can often be felt within the tip of the vermiform appendix which is then excised with a scalpel blade. The ram is allowed to stand, when a continuous flow of approximately 500 mL of urine is often produced. The ram must be carefully observed for normal urination and appetite.

iii. BUN and creatinine determinations, ultrasonography of the bladder and right kidney could be undertaken but are not necessary in this case because of the short duration of illness and resolution of the problem after amputation of the vermiform appendix.

iv. Early recognition of partial/complete urethral obstruction is essential because irreversible hydronephrosis develops rapidly due to the back pressure within the urinary tract. Reblockage with further calculi is possible. Surgical correction of urolithiasis involves a subischial urethrostomy under caudal block but is not a simple procedure and is undertaken only as a salvage procedure.

v. Control of urolithiasis involves feeding a correct ration with low magnesium content. The salt concentration of the ration can be increased to increase water intake. Urine acidifiers such as ammonium chloride can also be added to the ration. Good quality roughage should be available *ad libitum*.

217 In mid-spring you are presented with a 2-year-old Lleyn
ewe showing seizure activity
(217a). The sheep has drooping
of the left ear and lowered left
upper eyelid (ptosis). The sheep
appeared normal last evening.
There is lack of menace response
in the left eye and a flaccid left
cheek.
i. What conditions would you
consider? (Most likely first.)
ii. What laboratory tests could be undertaken to confirm your provisional
diagnosis?
iii. What treatments would you administer?
iv. What is the prognosis?

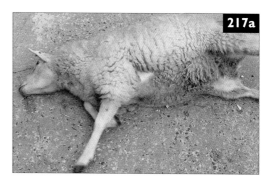

218 Severe lameness is reported affecting
2–5% of a group of 150 store lambs in
mid-autumn. Typically, only one claw of
one foot is affected. In all lambs there is
separation of the hoof capsule of the
lateral claw around the entire circum-
ference of the coronary band with some
regrowth of healthy horn at the coronary
band horn (218). The underlying corium
has a healthy smooth epithelium which
does not bleed. On the medial claw the
regrowth of healthy horn from the coronary band has progressed half-way down
the dorsal wall with the hoof capsule
thimbled at the toe. There is no associated
foul smell. There are several maggots

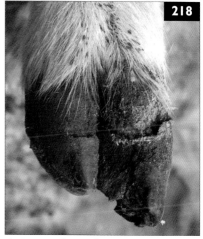

(myiasis) between the corium and hoof capsule in one foot of one lamb. In some
lambs there is interdigital infection with hyperaemia, swelling, and moistening of
the interdigital skin.
i. What conditions would you consider?
ii. What is the likely cause?
iii. What action would you take?
iv. How could this condition be prevented?

217 i. The most likely conditions to consider include: acute listerial meningoencephalitis; polioencephalomalacia; peripheral vestibular lesion with trauma to the left superficial facial nerve; acute coenurosis; sarcocystosis. Some cases of listeriosis can present with predominantly signs of acute meningitis rather than the more usual unilateral cranial nerve signs and obtunded mental state.

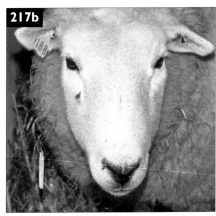

ii. Listeriosis can be confirmed following collection of lumbar CSF but this is not a simple procedure when the sheep shows seizure activity. An elevated protein concentration of 1–4 g/L (0.1–0.4 g/dL) (normal <0.4 g/L, <0.04 g/dL) and an increased white cell concentration (pleocytosis) with predominance of monocytes is typical of listeriosis.

iii. *Listeria monocytogenes* is susceptible to various antibiotics including penicillin (up to 300,000 IU/kg on day 1), ceftiofur, erythromycin, and trimethoprim/sulphonamide. Emphasis should be placed on administering the maximum dose of penicillin costs will permit at the first visit rather than the duration of daily penicillin injections thereafter. A single intravenous injection of soluble corticosteroid, such as dexamethasone at a dose rate of 1.1 mg/kg, may reduce the associated inflammatory reaction and improve prognosis. Sedation is rarely employed.

iv. It is difficult to afford an accurate prognosis and all cases should be treated aggressively. Despite the dramatic clinical signs this ewe made a good recovery and is shown 3 days later (**217b**).

218 i. The most likely conditions to consider include: contagious ovine digital dermatitis; virulent footrot; white line abscess.

ii. Contagious ovine digital dermatitis is the most likely cause of lesions originating at the coronary band. There is no ready explanation why only one foot is affected.

iii. All affected lame lambs should be isolated. All under-run horn is carefully removed then the foot sprayed with oxytetracycline aerosol. All lame lambs are given a single injection of long-acting oxytetracycline or tilmicosin.

iv. There are no specific control measures for contagious ovine digital dermatitis. Strict biosecurity should help prevent introduction of the disease. Prompt attention to all lame sheep should prevent such advanced painful lesions.

219 You are presented with a pedi-gree Suffolk ram which has been dull and inappetant for the past 7 days. The ram has a tucked-up abdomen consistent with a poor appetite. The ram often adopts a wide stance with the hindlimbs placed further back than normal and the head held lowered. There is frequent bruxism. Only a few drops of urine rather than a continuous flow are voided when

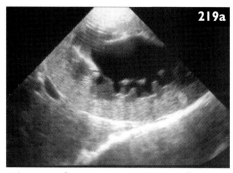

the ram urinates. The rectal temperature is normal (39.5°C (103.1°F)). The heart rate is increased at 90 beats per minute. The BUN concentration is elevated at 27.8 mmol/L (77.84 mg/dL) (normal range 2–6 mmol/L, 5.6–16.8 mg/dL). You suspect partial obstructive urolithiasis and scan the right sublumbar fossa with a 5.0 MHz sector transducer connected to a real-time, B-mode ultrasound machine.
i. Describe the sonogram shown in 219a.
ii. What action would you take?
iii. How could this problem have been prevented?

	1	2	3	4	5	6	7
Albumin g/L	33.1	28.3	12.5	13.1	24.1	25.1	22.5
(g/dL)	(3.31)	(2.83)	(1.25)	(1.31)	(2.41)	(2.51)	(2.25)
Globulin g/L	42.1	39.1	37.1	41.1	61.7	42.1	68.1
(g/dL)	(4.21)	(3.91)	(3.71)	(4.11)	(6.17)	(4.21)	(6.81)
Faecal worm							
egg count (epg)	100	200	250	6,000	100	150	150

220 Results of serum and faecal samples collected as part of a pre-liminary investigation of poor BCS in a group of six ewes (220) (sheep 2–7; sheep 1 is a normal control ewe) are presented above.

How would you interpret these findings?

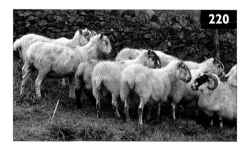

219 i. There is severe hydronephrosis with an enlarged fluid-distended renal pelvis and reduced renal medulla/ cortex (219b).

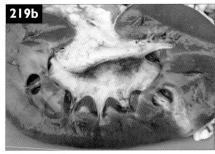

ii. Such renal pathology is irreversible and the ram should be euthanased for welfare reasons. Urethral obstruction results in bladder distension and back pressure causing hydroureter and hydronephrosis. The condition is bilateral and there is no requirement to scan the left kidney. Except for uroperitoneum in growing lambs, leakage from, or rupture of, the bladder is an uncommon event in adult sheep.

iii. Hydronephrosis is prevented by prompt identification of the sick ram by the shepherd with immediate veterinary attention to relieve the urinary tract obstruction.

Correct ration formulation with appropriate mineral supplementation (low magnesium) is the basis for prevention of urolithiasis in intensively reared sheep. Fresh clean water must always be available.

220 Sheep 1 has normal serum albumin and globulin concentrations >30 g/L (>3 g/dL) and 35–45 g/L (3.5–4.5 g/dL), respectively.

Sheep 2 has a serum protein profile typically observed in emaciated ewes without obvious bacterial infection or parasite infestation. Causes include poor molar dentition, lameness, and so on.

Sheep with a protein-losing enteropathy, notably paratuberculosis (very common; sheep 3 and 4) and nephropathy (rare), have profound hypoalbuminaemia (serum concentration <15 g/L, <1.5 g/dL) and a normal globulin concentration. Due to immunosuppression, sheep with paratuberculosis often have high faecal egg counts (>1,000 epg; sheep 4) resulting from increased fecundity of those mature nematodes present; diarrhoea is uncommon. It is exceptional for serum albumin concentrations to fall so low in cases of chronic intestinal parasitism such as haemonchosis.

Chronic severe bacterial infections (sheep 5) causing weight loss/ill-thrift result in significant increases in serum globulin concentration (often >55 g/L, >5.5 g/dL) and low serum albumin concentration (18–25 g/L, 1.8–2.5 g/dL).

If fed marginal protein levels during late gestation, serum albumin concentrations can fall as immunoglobulins accumulate in colostrum (sheep 6).

Subacute fasciolosis (sheep 7) results in hypoalbuminaemia, with increased serum globulin concentrations, often exceeding 65 g/L (6.5 g/dL). Further specific tests can then be selected based upon the organ system, e.g. serum GLDH and GGT concentrations and faecal fluke egg count for fasciolosis.

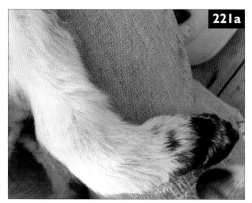

221 A 2-day-old 4.5 kg Greyface ewe lamb presents with a displaced fracture of the third metatarsal bone (221a).
i. How would you achieve effective analgesia for fracture realignment and repair?
ii. How would you repair the fracture?
iii. What other treatments would you recommend?

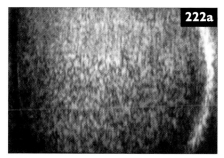 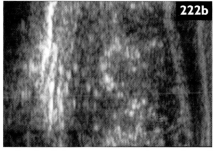

222 The sonograms (222a and 222b) were obtained from two recently purchased rams using a 5.0 MHz linear transducer connected to a real-time, B-mode ultrasound machine.
i. Describe the sonograms (both testicles similar in each ram).
ii. What simple selection criterion could farmers adopt at ram sales?
iii. What further fertility assessment(s) could be undertaken on ram 1?
iv. What advice would you offer?

221 i. Effective analgesia for fracture realignment and repair can be achieved after intravenous injection of a NSAID before the procedure. There are no injectable general anaesthetic drugs licensed for use in sheep in many countries but alphaxalone/alphadolone and propofol work very well. However, effective analgesia can be achieved immediately after lumbosacral extradural

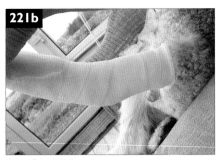

injection (15 mm 21-gauge needle) of 3 mg/kg of 2% lidocaine.
ii. The fracture is immobilized with a fibreglass cast (or similar) applied with slight flexion of the hock joint (**221b**). The hock angle maintains the cast in place while the cotton wool padding underneath permits growth over the next 3 weeks before removal. Simply applying traction to the distal limb without limb paralysis to effect reduction is cruel, largely ineffective, and results in overextension of the hock with straightening of the leg and loss of the plaster cast within hours/days (or the cast is applied too tightly).
iii. There is always the risk of bacteraemia in ruminants. A 10–14-day course of antibiotics is therefore indicated as a precaution against infection of the traumatized (fracture) site, but this instruction is rarely followed by the farmer.

222 i. The testicle from ram 1 has a uniform sonographic appearance and normal >7 cm diameter. The testicle from ram 2 is only 5 cm diameter, appears more hypoechoic than normal, and contains many hyperechoic spots. These hyperechoic dots are thought to represent the fibrous supporting architecture now more obvious due to atrophy of the seminiferous tubules. These findings are consistent with testicular atrophy.
ii. Farmers should measure the maximum scrotal circumference of all potential ram purchases using a tape measure, with acceptable values >36 cm for shearlings and >32 cm for ram lambs.
iii. Fertility assessment by semen collection and examination, whether by electroejaculation or artificial vagina, could be carried out on ram 1. A single semen sample would not indicate serving capacity. This is unnecessary for ram 2 because of the obvious testicular atrophy.
iv. Ram 2 should not be used for breeding for at least 3 months and must be reexamined before turnout with ewes. Without a more detailed history of the ram (previous illness), it is not possible to advise whether it would be worthwhile keeping the ram 1 more year until the next breeding season.

223 In spring you are presented with an obtunded 2-year-old Grey-face ewe. The sheep shows drooping of the left ear, deviated muzzle towards the right side, flaccid left lip, and lowered left upper eyelid (ptosis) (223a). There is lack of menace response in the left eye and profuse salivation with a flaccid left cheek with impacted food material.

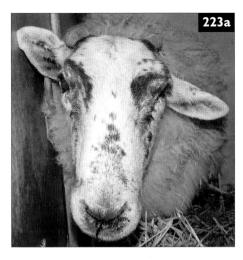

i. What conditions would you consider? (Most likely first.)
ii. What laboratory tests could be undertaken to confirm your provisional diagnosis?
iii. What treatments would you administer?
iv. What control measures would you recommend?

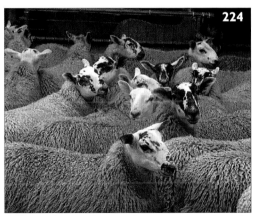

224 A commercial sheep client who purchases 280 yearling female replacements and 10 rams at auction sale every year is concerned about the flock's health status and asks your advice regarding potential problems arising from introduced stock (224).
i. What diseases could be introduced on to his farm? (Most economically important first.)
ii. What basic control measures could be adopted for the more important diseases?

223 i. The most likely conditions to consider include: listeriosis; OPT with trauma to the left superficial facial nerve; peripheral vestibular lesion with trauma to the left superficial facial nerve; brain abscess; acute coenurosis; sarcocystosis.

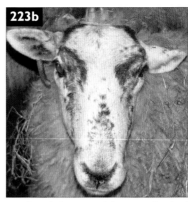

ii. Gross inspection of lumbar CSF collected under local anaesthesia using a 19-gauge 40 mm hypodermic needle (75–85 kg ewe) reveals no abnormality in cases of listeriosis. Laboratory examination reveals an elevated protein concentration of 1–4 g/L (0.1–0.4 g/dL) (normal <0.4 g/L, <0.04 g/dL), and a slight increase in white cell concentration (pleocytosis) comprised of large mononuclear cells.

iii. *Listeria monocytogenes* is susceptible to various antibiotics including penicillin (up to 300,000 IU/kg), ceftiofur, erythromycin, and trimethoprim/sulphonamide. A single intravenous injection of soluble corticosteroid, such as dexamethasone at a dose rate of 1.1 mg/kg, will reduce the associated severe inflammatory reaction and improve prognosis. The ewe is shown 2 weeks after treatment commenced in **223b**.

iv. Control involves correct fermentation of grass silage through the use of additives and air-tight storage. When feeding, discard all spoiled silage, clean troughs daily, and discard refusals.

224 i. Diseases which could be introduced include:
- Multiple-anthelmintic-resistant nematode strains (*Haemonchus contortus* and *Teladosagia* spp. in particular).
- *Psoroptes ovis* (sheep scab, including pyrethroid-resistant strains).
- *Chlamydophila psittaci* (EAE).
- Virulent footrot.
- Contagious ovine digital dermatitis.
- *Fasciola hepatica* (liver fluke).
- SPA (jaagsiekte).
- Orf (CPD).
- Paratuberculosis (Johne's disease).
- *Campylobacter fetus fetus.*
- Border disease.
- Pediculosis (lice).
- Scrapie (homozygous genotype for shortened incubation period).
- MVV.
- CLA.
- *Melophagus ovinus* (keds).

ii. Stock should be bought from a regular source with proven health status. All purchased sheep must be treated with an appropriate macrocyclic lactone preparation and levamisole upon arrival and left in the handling pens overnight to prevent pasture contamination. Careful inspection for ectoparasites is essential as macrocyclic lactone preparations do not kill lice and under certain situations plunge dipping may be a more appropriate treatment option. The sheep must be maintained in strict quarantine for at least 1 month after arrival on the farm.

The availability of a highly efficacious chlamydial abortion vaccine questions whether a large financial premium is justified for breeding female replacements from EAE-monitored flocks.

Any lame sheep should be carefully inspected. Serological screening against MVV infection is possible but seroconversion takes many months to develop and false-negative results may be obtained, especially in young sheep.

There is no serological screening test available for jaagsiekte. Some control of spread of jaagsiekte can be effected by maintaining sheep in age groups especially during housed periods. Screening for Johne's disease is not a practical option.

Selection based upon ram PrP genotype is unnecessary in commercial flocks producing lambs for slaughter.

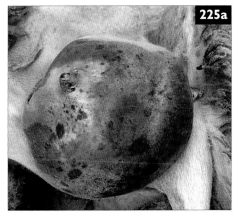

225 A two-crop ewe at pasture with month-old twin lambs at foot is found isolated from the remainder of the flock. The ewe appears very stiff and drags the left hindleg. The ewe is profoundly depressed with toxic mucous membranes. The rectal temperature is elevated (40.6°C (105.1°F)). The pulse is increased to 120 beats per minute. The respiratory rate is increased to 45 breaths per minute. There are no ruminal sounds. Examination of the udder reveals extensive gangrenous mastitis of the left gland with subcutaneous oedema extending along the ventral abdominal wall to the brisket (225a).
i. What pathogens could be involved?
ii. What is the prognosis?
iii. What would you recommend?
iv. What control measures could be adopted?

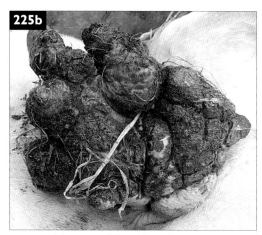

225 i. Gangrenous mastitis caused by *Mannheimia* spp. and *Staphylococcus aureus* occurs sporadically during the first 3 months of lactation associated with poor milk supply related to ewe undernutrition and overvigorous sucking by the lambs.

ii. Despite antibiotic and supportive therapy the prognosis is grave, and gangrenous udder tissue eventually sloughs leaving a large granulating surface with superficial bacterial infection. The granulation tissue continues to proliferate (**225b**) over the coming months (up to 10–20 cm diameter).

iii. These ewes are unsuitable for breeding stock. The infected granulation tissue and resultant drainage lymph node enlargement would result in carcass condemnation (and raise genuine welfare concerns). The fleece is very poor because growth has occurred during this period of illness and debility. The ewe should be euthanased for welfare reasons at first presentation.

iv. Control measures include ensuring ewes are well fed. Concentrates should be supplied to ewes and lambs when pasture is poor. No ewe should be expected to rear triplets. Teat lesions should be identified and treated with topical antibiotics.

Reading List

General texts which the reader may find useful:

Aitken I (ed) (2007). *Diseases of Sheep*, 4th edn. Blackwell Publishing, Oxford.

Andrews AH, Blowey RW, Boyd H, Eddy RG (eds) (2004). *Bovine Medicine: Diseases and Husbandry of Cattle*, 2nd edn. Blackwell Publishing, Oxford.

Ball PJH, Peters AR (2004). *Reproduction in Cattle*, 3rd edn. Blackwell Publishing, Oxford.

Divers T, Peek S (eds) (2007). *Rebhun's Diseases of Dairy Cattle*, 2nd edn. Elsevier, Amsterdam.

Maxie MG (ed) (2007). *Jubb, Kennedy and Palmer's Pathology of Domestic Animals (Volumes 1–3)*, 5th edn. Saunders, Philadelphia.

Radostits OM (2001). *Herd Health: Food Animal Production Medicine*, 3rd edn. Saunders, Philadelphia.

Radostits OM, Gay C, Hinchcliff KC, Constable PD (2007). *Veterinary Medicine: A Textbook of the Diseases of Cattle, Horses, Sheep, Pigs, and Goats*, 10th edn. Saunders, Philadelphia.

Scott PR (2007). *Sheep Medicine*. Manson Publishing, London.

Smith, BP (ed) (2008). *Large Animal Internal Medicine*, 4th edn. Mosby, New York.

Index: Cattle

Index: Cattle

Index: Sheep

Index: Sheep